My Exciting Cancer Journey

From a Death Sentence to The Great Wall of China

MARTYN HOPKINS

This edition first published 2021
Copyright Martyn Hopkins 2021

The right of Martyn Hopkins to be identified as the Author of this work has been asserted in accordance with the Copyrights, Designs and Patents Act 1988

All rights reserved. No part of this book may be reprinted or reproduced or utilised in any form or by any electronic, mechanical or other means, now known or hereafter invented, including photocopying and recording, or in any information storage or retrieval system, without the permission in writing from the Publishers.

ISBN 978-1-008-98014-3

DISCLAIMER

The author is not medically qualified and is not offering medical advice.

Cancer is a very serious illness and if you have, or suspect you might have, any of the illnesses or symptoms mentioned in this book, the author strongly recommends that you seek medical advice from a qualified medical practitioner.

This book is the author's account of his own experience and should you choose to follow any of the treatments discussed in this book, you should satisfy yourself that it is the right thing for you to do as the author accepts no responsibility for any outcomes.

INTRODUCTION

Martyn Hopkins was diagnosed in June 2018 with incurable stage 4 metastatic Prostate Cancer of the rare, aggressive and deadly Ductal Adenocarcinoma variant. Of approximately 48,000 Prostate Cancer diagnoses each year in Britain, only around 400 are of Ductal Adenocarcinoma.

Tumours and lesions had already spread to the spine, pelvis, left hip and lymph nodes and with a PSA score of 500 and a Gleason score of 8 (4+4) the odds were stacked against him. He was given 3-5 years to live – if he accepted everything the NHS could offer.

Along the way, he lost several friends to various cancers, at least one of them killed by Chemotherapy, and became frustrated at the complacency with which he was faced in the medical profession and their far too easy resignation to people dying.

But Martyn was not prepared to die simply because this disease and the NHS said he would, so he immediately started an aggressive campaign of research to find a treatment for himself that would defy the odds. What he found is treatments that can help anyone, no matter how much money they have and no matter the cancer or the progression of it, and has now made it his mission to share this information.

This is the story of how, with Martyn's research and an incredible family behind him, he was able to go for treatment to China and have CIK immunotherapy – a ground-breaking scientific innovation that sets the body's own immune system against the cancer with dramatic and decisive effect.

But along the way, Martyn poses the difficult questions about why cancer sufferers like him in Britain are left so far behind the curve and with treatments that themselves cause considerable suffering and cannot save the patient but only postpone dying.

With a wicked mix of humour and excoriating observation, he shines the light on what is wrong with cancer treatments in Britain whilst giving hope to cancer sufferers that a cure may be within their grasp – *even if they do not have the money to go to China for treatment.*

DEDICATION

This book is dedicated to my amazing family, to the love of my life, my wife, Sheena, who has been a rock; to my daughter, Eliza who set the crowd-funding in place and to my son Alex who threw his weight behind everything to make it happen as well as their respective wonderful spouses, Aymeric and Emma whose unstinting love and efforts helped to make it all possible, and to my beautiful Grandson Vincent who came along a little later but, just by being there and being himself has added sparkle and colour to all our lives as well as, for me, a very deep appreciation of what it means to have the privilege of still being around to have the chance to know him and love him.

I also dedicate it to my amazing wider family and friends (credited by name at the end) for their love, and for their fantastic efforts which combined to make my two incredible trips to China possible.

I also dedicate it to my Chinese Doctors, especially Dr Zhao Yuliang, Dr Nelson Dhu and Dr Yu Tao who took wonderful care of me and used skills and knowledge that, sadly, still have to come into use in the NHS. Also my Chinese nurses, especially Nancy, but all of the others too (too many to name) whose skilful care and unstinting cheerfulness helped to brighten our stay, and of course Cathy Wang who, incredibly, made it all fun with her sunny nature, her extensive knowledge of everything and her never-ending willingness to go the extra mile for us. The rest of the Chinese team also, especially Crystal, my very helpful and efficient first point of contact and all the others too many to mention by name but from radiographers to admin to cleaners, I thank you all.

Finally, to Macmillan who are astonishingly brilliant and supportive, as well as my oncology team in the UK and my outstanding General Practioner who spotted what was happening quickly.

CONTENTS

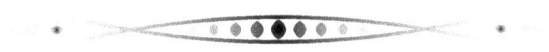

Chapter 1: Who Am I? 1
Chapter 2: How do you react to a Cancer Diagnosis?...........10
Chapter 3: The Scan and Biopsy Merry-go-round 22
Chapter 4: Worse news and the consequences.......................29
Chapter 5: Research 34
Chapter 6: The search for treatment 39
Chapter 7: Crowdfunding and my amazing family.................44
Chapter 8: China – First sights 47
Chapter 9: Treatment begins...54
Chapter 10: Tiananmen Square and Forbidden City................60
Chapter 11: Pattern of hospital life emerges.....................68
Chapter 12: On the scans merry-go-round – again!.............72
Chapter 13: Silk Street and Western Cakes! 90
Chapter 14: Cryosurgery refund 95
Chapter 15: Grand Opera - Chinese style 99
Chapter 16: The Great Wall of China.............................101
Chapter 17: CIK Day approaches 107
Chapter 18: Winding down...113
Chapter 19: Homeward bound.....................................117
Chapter 20: Why can you not get this in the NHS?............120
Chapter 21: What about other treatments? 130
Chapter 22: Back to the future....................................134
Chapter 23: Epilogue...146

Appendix 1...157
Appendix 2...160
Footnote – April 2021..162

CHAPTER 1

Who Am I?

I grew up in England in a loving working-class family in the New Town of Hemel Hempstead with my mother and father and an older sister. Mum & dad met in Scotland at Drem airfield during WWII when they both served in the Air Force, mum in the WAAF and dad as a Sergeant in the RAF.

Dad was a clever and resourceful man, he had been in the groundcrew in the RAF and variously worked on Bristol Beaufighters (undoubtedly his favourite aircraft) as well as Supermarine Spitfires and De Havilland Mosquitoes whilst with 96 Squadron, whose motto "We prowl by night" was apparently very well deserved and not only for their prowess with night fighter aircraft!

Like "Unc" in Only Fools and Horses, he had hundreds of stories that began with "During the war…" I loved his stories – mum didn't.

Mum was most often a housewife along with most of the ladies in our street but sometimes worked as a dinner lady at the nearby schools or in the accounts department at the Ovaltine factory in Abbotts Langley, or at the John Dickinson paper mills in Apsley. She was hard working and always maintained an impeccable house and impeccably turned-out kids. We were brought up with a strong Christian faith, which I still practice.

They were also extremely sociable and as a result we had lots of parties. Dad was a dab hand at "magic" tricks both for kids and for adults. Pushing a silver sixpence through the wall was a favourite for the kids and it is fairly obvious (with mum as accomplice) how he did that. One of my favourites that always caused astonishment was having an unpeeled banana that, after the required hocus pocus and getting the kids to shout "abracadabra", was peeled and found to be, "magically", cut into the same number of pieces as the kids at the party. I do know how to do this one after happening upon dad preparing for it once.

But some of his tricks were truly amazing - take for example, one that still mystifies me: He took a pack of cards and got one of the adults in his audience to choose a card from the pack. He then got them to sign their name on the front of the card. With the card put back into the pack, he then did lots of hocus pocus which culminated in him throwing the pack of cards in the air (and the kids shouting abracadabra of course) and then getting the kids to pick them all up and count them. We found that there were only 51 cards. Guess which one was missing. That's right, the signed one. But the punchline was that he asked the person that picked and signed the card if he had his car keys. "Yes" he said, "they are in my pocket". He withdrew said keys, and dad announced with a flourish "Go and open your car and the card is face down on the driver's seat". The whole audience trooped out to the car and was incredulous as the owner assured everyone the car had been locked throughout and that this was impossible. Nobody had either gone near dad or left the room during this performance (not that I had seen anyway – *and I was looking as I had seen variants of this trick before*), yet the card was there! Good old dad!

He always promised to tell me how to do this trick when I was 21. Unfortunately, it was not until I was older that I remembered to ask him again and he simply repeated that he would tell me when I was 21! Sadly, he took his secret to the grave.

Mum and dad had moved to Hemel Hempstead from Littlehampton when I was a few months old as dad had got a job at Rotax, an engineering firm set up mainly to service aircraft parts, and he got his job as an aero engineer there due to his RAF training. I can still remember the smell of the factory and how exciting it was to me to go round it with dad. He was a genial, cheerful and even-tempered man with a wicked sense of humour and a laugh like Mutley which I inherited. He was always ready with a joke. Everyone loved him.

I remember my childhood as very happy even though as a family we never had much money, but my sister and I did not go without much.

Born in January 1955 I was a "Baby Boomer" and I went to Bennetts End Secondary Modern School despite the fact that I was, in adulthood, found to have an above average IQ. I had deliberately flunked my 11+ exam so I could stay with my mates rather than go to the Grammar School but, even then I only missed a pass by a few marks, to the extent that mum tried (and failed) to get them to let me go to the Grammar anyway! This episode was undoubtedly my first, but not my last, somewhat less than brilliant decision as you'll see.

The Grammar School was in the same grounds as the Secondary Modern School. The two schools eventually merged to become Longdean Comprehensive School while I was still there as a 15-year-old in 1970. The Secondary Modern school buildings are now gone.

You'll probably think I am a crazy man calling my Cancer journey exciting but let me explain some things to you at the outset as a kind of backdrop to the rest of my story.

Firstly, nobody sane wants to get cancer and I am not, as far as I am aware, insane – I suppose it is possible to be insane and not be aware of the fact, but I do not believe myself to be insane.

Secondly, I have inherited from dad, an irrepressible and eclectic sense of humour often coupled with what my family call a dark side. My humour covers the whole range from light to dark, sometimes very dark, even black humour, but often strays into other areas that I would describe as mischievous rather than anything else. Usually, my humour is word-play – more than just simple puns but based on the use of words and their meanings. My schoolteachers recognised this and it sometimes cropped up, unfavourably, in my school reports – one notable comment as follows: "Martyn would be very good at English if only he would curb his sense of the ridiculous!" and another: "Martyn's role as the class clown is wearing thin!". Because of this sense of humour I am well able to enjoy laughing at myself and, trust me, there is often much to laugh at concerning me.

Still on the subject of humour and so you understand a little more about this and how it affects me, I love Blackadder, Only Fools and Horses and Fawlty Towers and always Robin Williams' humour – how the world misses him! So you get a glimpse into my preferred humour from this.

I am not so keen on what I call slapstick humour such as Laurel and Hardy, although I must admit the scene in Meet The Parents where the hapless Ben Stiller (AKA Greg (Gaylord) Fokker) who, having filled the garden where his future sister-in-law's wedding is to take place with the contents of the cesspit - *and* lost Robert DeNiro's (AKA Jack Byrnes) beloved cat Jinxy, is on the roof taking a crafty smoke in desperation at how badly his first weekend with his future in-laws is going. Jinxy happens by at this juncture and Greg makes a dive for him, disconnecting both the gutter which is full of leaves (to which he has set fire with his cigarette, which he dropped as he dived for Jinxy), and an electricity cable in the process, and all hell breaks loose. He has set in motion a chain of accidents which utterly destroys the garden setup including setting fire to and destroying a hand carved altar made by his fiancée's ex who clearly still has the hots for her! I find this scene screamingly funny, even though it is undoubtedly very firmly in the category of slapstick.

Thirdly, I love life. I love my family (especially my wife and soulmate, and my son and daughter and their amazing soulmates) and am utterly consumed with love and adoration for my little Grandson Vincent (after Van Gogh) who is without doubt, the most beautiful and intelligent little boy ever born in the history of mankind – and I am certainly not in any way biased in saying this, I assure you!

Fourthly, I love music – anything of quality, but take Opera for example, Tosca and Madame Butterfly amongst my favourites, and Luciano Pavarotti and Anna Netrebko are far and away my favourite Tenor and Soprano. I once took my wife to see Pavarotti in London's Hyde Park which was a truly magical experience. I also love classical music, Vaughan Williams' (The Lark Ascending transports me to an English meadow on a hot summer's day, especially when played by

Nigel Kennedy) and I am simply astonished that a man who saw such horrors in WWI could create such beauty. I also love Shostakovich (Piano Concerto No2 second movement Andante is pure genius) and if you have never listened to The Dance of the Knights by Prokofiev from Romeo & Juliet – do it - NOW! Yes – stop reading and go and find it, I promise you it will put you in the mood for excitement!

I love Rock music including, but not limited to, Yes; Led Zeppelin; Pink Floyd; Fleetwood Mac; Steely Dan (Yes, I know these cross musical Genres and are not simply "Rock" but I don't want you to fall asleep) and much, much more. Oh, and if you have not heard Robert Plant and Alison Krauss' Bluegrass album "Raising Sand" – it too is essential listening – play it after the Dance of the Knights – yes, that's right - the whole album.

Fifthly, I love speed, especially flying, and have flown (hands on the controls during some of the flight) in a Tiger Moth biplane and a WWII North American Harvard T9 (Texan) in which I was thrilled by a loop the loop and a barrel roll amongst other incredible aerobatics! I also love speed on the ground and have driven fast and very fast cars including proper racing cars, not competitively, but nevertheless serious racing cars – 2 litre turbocharged single seaters with slick tyres and wings – very, very fast – at speeds well in excess of 170mph according to the Marshalls with the speed gun at Mallory Park, a small race circuit in Leicestershire in case you don't know.

Sixthly, I love my garden, I love birds – in fact wildlife in general in fact creation in general including flora and fauna. We live in a beautiful world (despite some of our fellow custodian's best efforts to destroy it) and I have been privileged to travel to many countries – 19 different ones at the last count, many of them several times.

Seventhly, I love fine food, both eating and cooking. I am blessed with having not one but two chefs in my immediate family who have both worked at top 5* London restaurants including the Ritz, The London Hotel and the Dorchester and various private dining establishments such as The Gherkin and George – one of them (my son-in-law, Aymeric) a Sous Chef specialising in meat and fish and the other (my daughter, Eliza) a Patisserie Chef. From time to time they lavish their skills upon me. What bliss!!

Eighthly, in my career which, frankly, has not been a series of stellar successes but has at least been extremely varied and has also taken me to places I never expected to go, I started out as an apprentice cabinet maker. This after having turned down a place secured by Mr Boston, my Technical Drawing and careers teacher (and by far my favourite teacher), with a firm of architects who were going to put me through university and pay me for the privilege! I excelled at Technical Drawing (or Geometrical and Mechanical Drawing as it was then called) but I loved woodworking! Looking back this was certainly the second time I made what was far from the brightest decision I could have made.

I ended up being a kitchen fitter for my trouble! Still, along the way I got to work with some amazing people and make some lovely furniture and later on to fit some pretty nice kitchens in some pretty nice houses in and around London.

Later, I had an opportunity to join an Interior Design Practice where I became a partner. I enjoyed this hugely but clients can be odd (and worse) at times, like the one who, after having us design a Japanese bathroom for her stunning windmill property, complete with solid cedar bathtub and floor and cedar shoji screens, said she had decided against it in case she had a diarrhoea attack and it stained the floor!!!!! Or the client for whom we had created and installed three differently themed and very high quality bathrooms declared (face to face with me) that he thought we had done a brilliant job and they were delighted with it but, of the £11,000 outstanding he was only going to give me £3,500.00 because "How else do you think I made and kept my money – certainly not by giving it away and anyway – you must have heard of the "bash the subbie principle"?". He never did pay the remaining £7,500! As Blackadder would say – "Git!" Perhaps I should write a book about my experiences – now there's a thought - name and shame revenge! Ha, ha – I may just do that. Watch out you, so far, nameless of Barnet with a Polish surname beginning with "J" and ending "ski" – yes, that's right, you know who I mean!

This Interior Design business led onto being offered the UK distribution rights of a collection of high-quality woven fabrics from

Spain. This was great, except that the colour palette was a tough sell in northern Europe. If you have ever bought some fabric items or those little pottery wall ornaments on your Spanish holidays, you will know that they look great in the southern sun, don't they? But get them home to dear old Blighty and they look somehow – garish and out of place. Same problem with fabrics, colours that look great in southern Europe do not look so great in northern Europe due to the light. Nevertheless, I later seized an opportunity to snap up the sole UK distribution rights to a Swedish and German collection of very high-quality textiles and hand knotted wool rugs. This was amazing and was without the light issue, so it worked very well. The business was successful and built up quickly selling into hotels, cruise lines and the interior design markets but, sadly, I was ultimately and very reluctantly forced to sell the distribution rights back to the parent company and that was the end of that.

I went from there back to the kitchens industry as Head of Design and MD Designate of a company I had previously worked for, designing very high-end contemporary kitchens for companies such as the swanky London developers Candy & Candy. For long and complicated reasons involving the Department for Transport, an insurance company, and very highly paid lawyers – this very profitable company went bust so I joined a Maidenhead based kitchens company as Contracts Director but the company was in trouble from before I joined (although they hid this fact from me at my interviews) and I was made redundant just a year later. This company also no longer exists. I went from there to another high-end kitchens company in north London as a contracts manager. This position lasted five years during which time I oversaw the installation of some very nice kitchens indeed. I grew in my role in this company and later was also entrusted with some director level, and very successful, negotiations on behalf of our company with a very, very prestigious ultra-modern kitchens manufacturer in Italy called Minotti, during which I persuaded them to manufacture "own brand" kitchens for us – something they had always refused to do for anyone before. We started designing and selling ultra-high-end contemporary kitchens with stone door and drawer fronts and worktops etc. Truly beautiful.

However, this company too subsequently ran into problems for other reasons (beyond my control) and ultimately failed.

I was beginning to feel Like Jonah. They should have paid me not to join them!!

My final stint in kitchens was as a Project Manager - the one I was at when I received my cancer diagnosis while I was based in Barnes in West London (more on this later).

Somewhere in there, I also did two stints as Senior Clerk in Barrister's Chambers, starting in Lincoln's Inn in a position offered to me by a very dear friend and where I had a handful of Barristers in my charge. This was a commercial law set, specialising in insurance and reinsurance matters and immigration.

This Civil set later merged with a much larger Civil set in Holborn and I became Practice Manager there with some 60 Barristers in my charge. That was OK but subsequently this set absorbed a Criminal set from near the famous Old Bailey criminal courts. Now Commercial and Criminal law are two very, very different animals and clerking them is so different as to almost be two different professions. I knew nothing about criminal Barristers at all, except what I might have gleaned from TV adaptations of "Rumpole of the Bailey" and "Silk" both of which, whilst entertaining, I assure you do not offer any insight whatsoever into real criminal clerking matters!

In addition, the criminal set came with a very senior clerk and it soon became clear that he was going to assume complete control of the whole Chambers. I left, or rather was unceremoniously invited to leave by my joint Head of Chambers a very senior QC who thought he was something truly special, but he was so completely lacking in class and decency that he dismissed me by text message! Class is not conferred by letters after one's name, rather as my mother always used to say, "handsome is as handsome does". That's quite enough said about him, he is not worth the waste of another word – let alone the waste of an amusing Blackadder expletive.

I did a further and rather less notable stint as Senior Clerk, again brought about by my good friend, this time based in Piccadilly, but if I tell you that the owner of this Chambers along with one of the senior Barristers in Chambers were raided by the National

Crime Agency and had property, including an Hotel and a Bentley Mulsanne, confiscated on money laundering charges, you will see that this position was doomed from the start!

Shortly afterwards both I and my friend chose to leave for these reasons, and the set soon dissolved in disgrace! The story was in the national papers however but was, if nothing else, quite exciting! The Barrister concerned was late into Chambers one day saying that he had been held up having a new washing machine fitted. I asked if he had worn the old one out laundering his money? He had the grace to laugh, in fact he enjoyed the joke a lot!

Finally, my journey with cancer took me to places I never expected to go although I always *wanted* to go to some of these places, though by no means all of them. Some of these places are genuinely exciting and I hope you will see this from my descriptions.

If you understand the foregoing and see what I tell you in this narrative coloured against the backdrop of the foregoing, I believe you will understand me much better and also what I am trying to convey to you which is not simply that I had an unusual cancer treatment that saved my life but how and why I had it. With all the motivations I had to remain alive, and all the interesting experiences I have had, I simply refuse to die or even consider dying.

I felt rather like the artist, Cavaradossi, in the Opera, "Tosca" who, burning with love (and lust) for Tosca, is to be executed at the behest of the sadistic chief of police, Scarpia. The vicious Scarpia offers beautiful Tosca a Faustian bargain – to give herself to him and in return he will spare Cavaradossi's life. Grand drama indeed, leading to the night before Cavaradossi is due to die who, on the battlements of the prison, sings E Lucevan le Stelle (and the stars were bright) the climax of which roughly translates as - "I have to die, but I have never had so much reason to live". Sung by Pavarotti – this is just so exquisitely plaintive and painful – check it out.

In essence, this was me – I had so many reasons to live but had been told, in no uncertain terms, that I was to die.

So, to the nitty gritty and the main reason you purchased this book – my exciting cancer journey.

CHAPTER 2

How do you react to a Cancer Diagnosis?

I don't know how much the foregoing had a bearing on my initial reaction to my diagnosis, but I can honestly say I never felt the shock that many people speak of when receiving such a diagnosis. Now, I don't believe that this is because I am a tough cookie mentally or emotionally, actually I don't think I am. I cry at funerals for example – all funerals, even if I didn't know the person, but I suppose the judgement on whether or not I am a tough cookie is for others. I also honestly never ever had thoughts such as "why me?". I mean – why not me? It happens to so many men after all – why should I expect to dodge the bullet when so many other poor souls do not? That simply is not logical, so why waste time, effort and stress on wondering why it got me?

In cold hard figures, approximately 1 in 8 men will get Prostate Cancer (currently around 48,000 a year in the UK)[1] and of those less than 1% (under 400) will get the type I have - Ductal Adenocarcinoma, so I joined a fairly exclusive club, not that I would have joined given the choice. As Groucho Marx said "I would never join a club that would have me as a member!".

---

[1] Cancer Research UK – online 2020

Currently, almost 12,000 die in the UK each year of Prostate Cancer[2] – a quarter of those diagnosed – every year! The grim reaper has indeed found a bountiful field to harvest and he does it with disturbing enthusiasm.

According to my Oncologist, there is not much research into Ductal Adenocarcinoma as there are so few patients with it and the resource is therefore concentrated on the greater number which, although perhaps unfortunate for me, makes some sort of sense I suppose – *although*……. what if the key to understanding *all cancers*, lies in understanding Ductal Adenocarcinoma? Now there's something to ponder in idle moments!

Ductal Adenocarcinoma is so named (I had to know so I asked) because of the shape of the tumours and not for any other reason according to my Oncologist.

So, my dear friend – my Brother in Arms, as I shall now call you, if you are unfortunate enough to be a member of the same club, whichever branch of it you have joined – or been conscripted into, the basic level that the general hoi polloi get or the more exclusive Ductal Adenocarcinoma membership, or any other cancer for that matter that has metastasised to stage 4 as in my case then, as I see it you have three options:

1. Give up mentally. You will surely die and it will be soon, regardless of any medication you may choose to accept.
2. Accept and trust what the NHS can offer you which, for the most part, they give to you in good faith, believing it to be the best medical science can offer. You will surely die, but slowly. Maybe 5-10 years, average 7 years, and your quality of life will at times be, frankly, abject.
3. You can fight. You can research and you can find treatments that will, with a little luck, cure your cancer (Yes, I said cure it – but understand nothing is guaranteed on this journey) If nothing else it could at least buy you very much more time and a far better quality of life on your way. The

---

[2] Cancer Research UK – online 2020

fact that you are reading this, suggests that you have already chosen option 3. If so, Good for you – I am proud of you! If you have not made your mind up yet, then read on and please think about what you read very carefully. I truly hope it will both save you a lot of time and help you decide what to do and, perhaps it will also save your life.

If, in your case, there is no metastasis, in other words the cancer is contained in the Prostate itself, then you have other NHS options open to you. Brachytherapy for one, where they seed the tumour with radioactive "seeds" which kill it from within, and/or radiotherapy. You will also have options with other cancers than Prostate.

They may also offer surgery, hormone treatment, chemo and/or radiotherapy. Beware though, survival rates are measured in the average life expectancy of the patient disregarding quality of life. However, in my view, even leaving out quality of life issues, the published survival rates still do not make happy reading. Still, I know some who have had, and are having, these various treatments and who currently appear alive and well, and several for far more than 10 years, so you may wish to consider and/or go for one or more of these and I do not disparage you in the slightest for that. Nevertheless, my story may still help you as some of the treatments discussed will work on cancer that is contained in the prostate and will indeed have a very much higher prospect of a cure. Read on please.

The same choices are true for more or less any type of metastasised cancer as previously stated, but this book is based on Prostate Cancer, although I hope it may help with other forms of this vicious disease that is so rampant now.

So, my story, and the reason for this book, concerns primarily Stage 4 Metastatic Prostate Cancer, in my case variant Ductal Adenocarcinoma, with which I was diagnosed in June 2018. The death sentence from my title.

Looking back, in my case it began as I guess most men's experience of Prostate Cancer begins. Getting up in the night to pee, and gradually this increases in both frequency and in urgency.

I also had other symptoms such as unpleasant sensations in the penis and groin area, increasingly severe lower back pain, excessive and increasing fatigue and increasing ED.

Personally, I put night-time peeing down to my age. After all, we hear of this as a problem that comes with advancing age. This, along with an increasing problem with ED. Frankly, both are a miserable experience, but here I was, somewhat overweight (officially obese which is a hideous term), stressed with my work as a project manager for the very high-end kitchens and bedrooms company in London, and getting older. I was *expecting* to feel these issues to be honest, or at least was not surprised to be experiencing them. After all, I had tried several gym memberships and various weight loss diets with good intentions but, frankly, I lacked the motivation to keep going with either. It is just so tedious running or rowing on a machine or side training or static cycling, or living on foods you don't particularly enjoy - I can't bear it.

I had a daily commute on the train or by car from West London at the end of the Piccadilly Line into Hammersmith and from there to Barnes where I was based, by bus. In addition, I also often had to go into central London to visit sites, which I always did on the bus and tube.

Whether I travelled by car or by tube to my office, the journey was an hour, so usually I opted for car as it was a company car and my parking was paid for. By the time I got home in the evenings, I was knackered and wanted nothing more than to cook something nice to eat and relax for the evening in front of the telly. So, nice food, often a nice wine and "veg-ing" out on the sofa. What else can you expect but to put on weight and become rather less than completely healthy?

You may though, dear Brother in Arms, be wondering why I tolerated these somewhat distressing symptoms? The truth is, I did not simply tolerate them. I sought out every possible remedy for the ED – at the time the more distressing of the two symptoms, and these remedies tended to work for a while and then stop. I even resorted to finding herbal and other methods of increasing my testosterone level and, to be fair, they worked to some extent but it turned out to be a

"Big mistake – big - huge" (to quote Julia Roberts to a shocked sales assistant in the film Pretty Woman. The sales assistant had refused to serve her in a swanky ladies clothing store because she was dressed like a streetwalker (which she was) only for her to return the next day looking like – well - a very expensively dressed and glamorous Julia Roberts, laden with numerous bags stuffed with many, many thousands of dollars' worth of yet more expensive clothes, paid for by Richard Gere, from other Rodeo Drive stores which she showed off to the crestfallen sales assistant who, as Ms Roberts gleefully and spitefully pointed out, was paid on commission.

In my case the big mistake was, not turning Julia Roberts away, but taking testosterone enhancing preparations because it turns out that Prostate Cancer feeds on testosterone so I was making the, as yet, unknown cancer problem worse by trying to make the ED problem better!

To make matters still worse, the body plays a vicious trick on you when you take these drugs and other remedies by letting the ED get better for a short time before getting worse again – presumably as the Prostate Cancer builds its appetite for the increasingly bountiful feast of testosterone with which it is now being blessed! So you take more. And more. And more. Until eventually it no longer works at all and finally it dawns on you that something more serious is wrong.

The problem is that, at a primal level, this is an attack on your manhood. I mean, getting an erection is something so inseparably masculine that if you cannot achieve it you feel as if in some way you are no longer a man. So, you look for explanations for it like – I'm stressed, I'm overweight, I'm tired, I'm this, I'm that because, after all, you are a man and men get erections! Have you ever seen the Cerne Abbas Giant? It is what he is famous for – a monster sized erection! Look him up online.

You are also unwilling to consider the possibility that this ED might be permanent or even the symptom of something terrible. Why? – because it can't be – can it? Yes, I know there are some potential ways around it – none of which are very appealing, perhaps the worst of which is injections directly into the Little General. WHAT???

– YOU HAVE TO BE KIDDING ME!!!! And, you expect me to perform after that? Who thought this up – a misandrist lesbian?

What about the "little blue pill" – Viagra, or the little yellow pill, Cialis?

At the very beginning, these worked too, but after a while they petered out in effectiveness. I tried taking two, but simply got monster headaches and blurred vision and no difference with the Honourable Member for Littlehampton. Anyway, ED was not my only, or even biggest, problem as it turned out.

Regarding the nocturnal micturition, or Nocturnal Polyuria, or simply Nocturia as it is variously called by doctors, there is a story to this that explains why I did not do something earlier. Bear with me for another story, there is a point to it….

Many years ago, I had what was called a stricture. The long and the short of that is that it is a physical blockage where the urethra joins the bladder and this makes it impossible to pee. Well it would – there is no longer a hole for the pee to travel through, so it is hermetically sealed into the bladder.

The irony is that it came on quite suddenly on FA Cup final day of 1985. I had a friend round to watch the cup final with me and naturally, being blokes, we indulged in a few beers.

Towards half time, I started to need to pee. When half time came, I dashed upstairs to the loo and breathed a sigh of relief as I pointed Percy at the Porcelain, only to discover I could not produce a drop. Not one single measly drop, no matter how hard I tried. Nothing, Nyet, Nada. Needless to say, I tried for some time to no avail whatsoever.

When finally, I gave up and resolved to wait it out until full time (quite how I would manage that I wasn't sure) I limped gingerly downstairs and sat uncomfortably to watch the second half – and extra time. Anyway, convinced it would all resolve itself in due course, I had another couple of beers – well it would have been rude not to wouldn't it?

The match frankly, didn't mean much to me, not being a fan of either of the protagonists and anyway by this time as I was squirming in my seat like a schoolboy that was scared to put his hand up to ask to go out to the toilet.

The cup final was not even the most riveting affair to a neutral, and it ended 1-0 to Manchester United after enduring Extra time as well – 120 minutes of total torture, both at a football level and even more because of my inability to pass water, and I am not sure I could have told you anything about the match. I was absolutely in agony and bursting to go. Still not a drop, not one.

My wife and mother-in-law came in around this time, and saw my distress. My Mother-in-law announced in an imperious tone that the remedy was water as beer blocks you up! Bless her, she meant well (I think).

By this time I was really getting panicky and was looking like I was 5 months pregnant. I decided to go to A&E at Bedford Hospital, near where I lived and, true to usual form in A&E was waiting for more than an hour and a half. In the end, I was in such agony and now looked 6 months pregnant (I was actually quite slim at this time with a svelte 36" waist, so the bump was very pronounced) that my wife, at this point, became angry and went and demanded attention for me (she is a formidable woman) whereupon I was taken to a cubicle and, to my blessed relief they put in a catheter through my belly button. My "pregnancy bump" went down before my eyes and what looked like, and probably was, two gallons of pee went into the receptacle.

Why, you might ask, am I telling you this shaggy dog story?

Because, what ensued was an operation (for which I am truly thankful to have been unconscious) during which an instrument was inserted (yes, that way!) and the stricture was removed.

A few weeks of bleeding in diminishing quantities followed and now, to my joy, when I went to Syphon the Python I could pee like an elephant, honestly it was like a fire hose, but the important thing – and the reason why I have told you this story, is that the surgeon told me after the surgery that, henceforth, I would always be susceptible to water infections.

Sure enough, perhaps every two to three years, I would get an infection and make a pilgrimage to my GP who would duly prescribe an antibiotic and the problem would go away until next time.

So, to tie this story in with the cancer issue, I was not alarmed in early March 2018 when I got what again, seemed like a water infection, albeit quite a severe one this time.

GP duly visited, antibiotics duly secured and problem apparently resolved within the expected few days.

From that fateful cup final day 1985, Fast forward thirty-three years to a couple of weeks after this latest water infection and my esteemed mother-in-law, (yes, the same one – I have only been married once) had booked for the extended family to have a long weekend away in a large country house near Skegness – all 21 of us. And it was great, we all enjoyed ourselves including having a talent contest in which all took part and which was riotously good fun. I played Bjorn in Abba along with my brother and sister-in-law Ian and Alison's Benny and Agnetha and my wife's Anni-Frid, but I also played Michael Parkinson interviewing my mother-in-law as Dame Edna Everidge, replete with lots of glitter and a pink/purple wig in which she did not make the slightest attempt at an Antipodean accent but instead delivered her lines in her strong East London accent which just made it funnier! She was certainly no ordinary superstar! What a hoot!

We also had a murder mystery which was great in this big country house. I was the designated victim and when I "died" I must have done it so convincingly that my two little great nephews thought it was real and would not stop cuddling me for the rest of the holiday – it was so sweet of them and very touching that they were so concerned for their uncle.

But my nocturnal sojourns to the toilet persisted and in fact were more frequent than recent times, although no discomfort was evident.

A week or so after we returned home, my water infection returned, so I returned to my GP, a truly lovely lady who always had time for me and never sat with her pen poised over her prescription pad, so to speak – (it is now all computerised of course). But she listened, thought about it, discussed it and only then diagnosed. After a test, there and then in the surgery, she announced that no infection appeared to be present but, given the success of the antibiotics in suppressing the symptoms at least, she would prescribe these again but wanted to arrange for me to have an urgent blood test. This she did. The antibiotics worked to a degree once again but not completely, so I knew something more was wrong.

I had the blood test a couple of days later and knew there was bigger trouble when the doctor called me the day after the test. She was very kind, and said "well, your liver and kidney functions are normal..........pause........ (my mind was instantly screaming "BUT WHAT??") ....but your PSA score is rather high".

I had not the foggiest idea what a PSA score is so, being me, I asked. She said, "It is Prostate Specific Antigen and your score is 441". I said "OK, if that is high, what should it be?" She said, "in a man of your age, it should not be higher than 3". I said, "do you mean 300?". She said "No, 3". "Oh", I said, "so at 438 points higher than that, it looks as if there might be a tiny problem?". She knew me well enough to be able to laugh which I found endearing.

The conversation went on for a bit but, essentially, knowing nothing about this subject, I did not have the tools to continue very far with it and in any event, she explained that there were several possible causes that were not necessarily cancer, but she wanted me to see a consultant by which, I subsequently found out, she meant a consultant urologist.

The Big C word was out there now. I clocked it and decided I had to read about PSA scores and what they mean.

Essentially, a PSA score above 3 in men of around this age is never good news, but it might not be terrible news. It can be caused by, for example, Prostatic Hyperplasia, which is an enlarged Prostate but not a cancerous one, or Parathyroid malfunction or inflammation of the Prostate or an injury to the Prostate and some other things. This can produce many of the same symptoms as cancer including a high PSA score. So, a PSA score is only an indicator and is not definitive in any way. Nevertheless a PSA score into the hundreds as mine was, or even the thousands, which is possible, is definitely bad news, but the question is, how bad?

So, I was glad when my hospital appointment came around.

Everything, you soon discover once you climb onto this particular treadmill with the NHS, takes 2 weeks. 2 weeks for an appointment, 2 weeks for a scan, 2 weeks for a "hello, how are you?". It is regarded as the Gold standard in the NHS, but not by me – for me it is the wooden spoon standard – it's just not good enough and smacks of complacency as it has become the norm – even the target.

The consultant was reading my notes when I entered the consulting room, but had clearly already read them as he knew quite a bit of my history which he could not have read in the few moments he took scanning them in front of me. I found this somewhat comforting.

After a few minutes of discussion about my symptoms he invited me into an examination room and announced that he wanted to perform a Digital Rectal Examination. This, I discovered, is not a scan with an electronic device - it is the dreaded "finger up the bum".

With some melodrama, he pulled on the latex glove and allowed it to make that sharp snapping noise with his middle finger extended. (Actually, I am not sure if that is really true or if my overactive imagination had taken over!). In my mind I saw the scene from Blackadder when the baby eating Bishop of Bath and Wells, with a red-hot poker in his hand, in a booming voice tells the indebted and impecunious Edmund "Bend over Blackadder!".

Anyway, what is certainly true is that he told me to lie on my side in the foetal position following which he slavered lubricant at the orifice in question and proceeded to slide his finger in.

Now this procedure is not painful, but it is deeply humiliating which in itself causes something akin to pain. However, it lasted all of three seconds after which he said "alright, that's enough, if you would like to get dressed and come back into my room……". Then he promptly disappeared through the door to the adjoining consulting room whence we had come.

Unfortunately, there were no tissues on hand in the examination room, so I had to get dressed with a squidgy, slippery feeling between my bum cheeks, which was definitely not pleasant.

However, I duly followed his instructions and when I arrived back in his office, the first thing I noticed was that there was now a nurse there with him.

"So", he announced, with little ceremony but due gravity in his voice, "I am 99.9% sure you have cancer, and given the size and location of the tumour, I am also sure it will have metastasised. Usually, these Prostate Cancers go the bones and soft tissues when they metastasise but we will run some scans and tests to see what is happening."

Then he said the only thing that seemed to me a bit scary "Please be careful about lifting anything and do not lift heavy weights at all because, if I am right and this has gone into your spine, it can make the bone brittle and if it breaks or collapses you could be paralysed!".

I said "Phew, I thought I was in trouble for a minute". I don't think he understood the joke. He certainly didn't laugh, or even smile. The nurse smiled weakly but looked at me as if she was expecting me to keel over or slip to the floor in a blubbering mess and was poised like an Olympic sprinter on the starting blocks ready to leap forward to break my fall.

I am actually a pretty calm sort of fellow and it struck me that he had not tried to sugar coat this at all. I rated his bedside manner at 3 out of 10. But, I mused, there is no easy way to tell someone this news so you may just as well come straight out with it.

Anyway, I must have been unusually calm since the nurse asked me several times if I was alright and each time, I assured her I was. Then she asked how I was getting home to which I said I would drive home as my car was in the car park. She seemed very concerned at this and asked if was sure I felt OK to drive. I supposed that she must see a whole range of reactions from tears to wailing to people becoming an amorphic jellylike mass. Perhaps someone being quite this calm was actually disconcerting *for her*, but to tell the truth I was really fine.

My shock level was probably about the level you would get if you return to your car to find a parking ticket on the windscreen when you knew you had overstayed the time you had paid for. Not really shock at all – more, sort of, pissed off about it.

At the end of the consultation, he said he would be arranging for me to have a bone scan as soon as possible.

So, leaving the clinic, I was genuinely not distraught or shocked, I didn't feel tearful or upset, I just thought, "OK well, what do we do about it?". I did notice I was walking very carefully as I made my way back to my car, not only because of the squidgy mess between my bum cheeks but in case I jolted my spine and fractured it – but this over-caution soon passed. I went home, had a shower and went to work.

So, I shortly received the appointment for the bone scan – 2 weeks.

CHAPTER 3

The Scan and Biopsy Merry-go-round

So, I arrived back in front of the Urologist 2 weeks after the scan who said "Unfortunately, the bone scan is inconclusive, so I am going to send you for a CT scan".

Being me, I asked him "What will a CT scan show that the bone scan didn't?". He said it would show what was going on in the bones more clearly! So what the hell is the point of a bone scan?? And….. given that he wanted the bone scan that, as he knew and as I now know, can be inconclusive, why oh why did he not order both at the same time??? 4 weeks wasted!!!

Anyway, off I toddled and awaited my scan and next appointment - 2 weeks and 2 weeks. This is where the penny dropped as to what I was getting into. I saw a tortuous round of Hospital appointments and scary treatments stretching out ahead of me.

By the way, in case you don't know, A CT scan is a Computerised Tomography scan. What it means is that it is a special type of X-ray using a scanner and computer equipment to make images of the affected area.

It differs from a standard X-ray insofar as it produces black and white images of cross-sections of, in this case, the spine and pelvis. The pictures look as if you have been cut in half and you are looking slice by slice at your insides heading from your tummy down to your groin. It is actually quite interesting in fact.

The CT machine is not particularly scary, it is like a large doughnut and you lie on a sliding bed which moves into the doughnut so the technicians (Radiographers) are able to move you in or out until you are in the right position. Once there, the scan proceeds without much fuss. They project pictures of furry animals and serene lake scenes or flowers and butterflies onto the ceiling and play soft music for those of a nervous disposition, which I am not – I asked if I could have Led Zeppelin on but they did not have any!

The appointed day came around for me to see the Consultant Urologist again 2 weeks later. My wife drove me there this time at her insistence. She too expected me to need assistance, I think.

We walked into his office which was darkened and I saw some images on his computer screen. The nurse was there again, so I now thought it must be really bad. You soon learn to spot the signs.

"Well", he said "these are the scans. If you look here...." He pointed to the screen and showed me a significant tumour in my L5 vertebra, a lesion on each side of my pelvis and one on my left hip. "It also shows your lymph nodes are enlarged due to cancer".

He said, "It is not as bad as I was expecting, normally these scans are lit up like a Christmas tree" and he proceeded to show me some other poor sod's scan showing exactly what he had described, the spine, pelvis and everything else lit up just as he said, like a Christmas tree and, looking at it, I thought this a very apt, if rather macabre, simile. It appealed to my dark side and I smiled.

I said "OK, let's cut to the chase then, if this is not bad, what do we do from here?".

He said "Well, I didn't say it's not *bad*, I said it is not *as bad as I was expecting*. You must understand, this *will* kill you – we cannot save your life, but we can buy you some time." (2 out of 10 for bedside manner this time).

I said "how much time?"

He advised that if I had all the treatments they could offer, I should live between 5-10 years with the average for someone in my condition being around 7 years.

I was 63 years old at the time and thought that 7 years probably wasn't so bad especially given that new treatments are coming all the time – I would accept those odds.

Anyway, he said he would make an appointment for me with an Oncologist.

So, my first appointment with my Oncologist (yes, 2 weeks later), a lady with a somewhat disconcerting habit of closing her eyes when speaking directly to you. I mean closing them and keeping them closed. I have never met anyone with this curious habit before, but she was very pleasant albeit that it is very hard to read her face because of it. I thought she'd be very good at Poker – as long as she could remember her cards and where to put her chips!

She reiterated what the Urologist had already told me but said she wanted me to have an MRI scan. For me, this Oncology appointment was a bit of a waste of time frankly, except in one respect: By this time I should say that I was getting considerable pain when doing number two's and she started me on Bicalutamide which is essentially, a hormone treatment designed to block the production of testosterone and prevent the cancer from feeding on the male hormone. The cancer shrinks as a result of this treatment.

This worked dramatically and in a matter of a few days completely stopped the pain when doing a poo, and it also reduced the number of times I had to get up in the night to pee, in fact for some considerable time I did not get up at all in the night. "I'll just stay on these" I thought but, apparently, they will stop working after a while and the cancer will escape the inhibiting effects of it, so it is only a temporary fix at best.

Back to the MRI:

Again, for those that do not know, an MRI scan is a Magnetic Resonance Imaging scan. It uses strong magnetic fields and radio waves to take pictures of the relevant areas. It again differs from a standard X-ray as it produces very detailed pictures of the target areas.

An MRI machine is a totally different animal to a CT machine. For those of a nervous disposition, honestly, it can present a challenge.

It has a similar sliding bed system to a CT scanner, but instead of the large doughnut there is a much smaller tube that they slide you into. This can feel very claustrophobic as the diameter of the tube is not much bigger than you, so the roof of the tube is literally a matter of a couple of inches or so from your nose. My strategy for dealing with it was to close my eyes and force myself to think of something else and lie very still so that nothing messed up the scan so as to cause them to have to do it again.

This is also challenging though because a scan can last 20 minutes or more during most of which time you are inside the tube. It is truly amazing how many itches you acquire when you can't move! It is also extremely noisy and sounds as if you are inside a cement mixer that is being cleaned with water and bricks in it (if you have ever seen this being done on building sites you will recognise the sounds) because at times it makes loud bangs and clattering and churning noises.

Oh and I forgot to mention that I had at various times for these scans, a ½ litre of Barium to drink to create better soft tissue contrast imaging and a radioactive marker injection for the same purpose.

If you are faced with these, my advice is to simply go with it – the Barium is a white liquid, not disgusting (though I would have preferred a Pina Colada) and the injection is just an injection except it is delivered from a lead covered syringe. Oh, and they warn you that yet another injection that you get when in the CT scanner itself might make you feel warm around your groin, give you a taste of metal or make you feel you need to pee. I only felt the warmth in the groin area and it was not entirely unpleasant, just strange.

The Oncologist also wanted me to have a Biopsy.

Well, the day of the Biopsy came around (2 weeks!), but I had no date for the MRI to be done.

Now, this is a bit graphic, my Brother in Arms, but you need to know so you can get yourself prepared. Nobody told me what was coming, but I wish they had.

Essentially, a biopsy on the Prostate Gland is firstly, not pleasant, and secondly quite risky. The risk is that you can get a very serious infection as they get to the Prostate via the colon, in fact they make a hole in the wall of the colon (colonic transection) and then access the Prostate with the instrument for taking the biopsy samples through this hole.

In preparation for this procedure, they stuff you with antibiotics including tablets to take the day before and different tablets to take on the day plus a pessary to shove up your bum an hour before arriving at the hospital.

Dark side alert: What if you live an hour and a half train journey from the hospital? I have a mental picture of a guy on the 7:15 from Birmingham New Street when, an hour from the hospital, tells his fellow passengers that he is going to make a pessary disappear before their very eyes and, dropping his trousers and pants, inserts the pessary and pulls his pants up again before saying to his horrified audience "and for my next trick…..")". Notice the dark side and sense of the ridiculous combined here!

Seriously though, the problem with this whole process is that you lose your dignity pretty early on and you become somewhat unconcerned about things that others would be mortified by, and indeed what you would have been mortified by yourself only a few weeks before. In the end, I suppose it is like a woman giving birth, so many people, both men and women, have had a look at her "down there" that she is not bothered anymore – "roll up, roll up, penny a look!".

Anyway, quite seriously now, if you are unfortunate enough to get an infection from a Prostate biopsy procedure, it could be extremely serious even dangerous (urinary tract infection, prostatitis, orchitis, bacteraemia, and sepsis among the potential problems. Sometimes, these complications are severe enough to lead to hospitalisation, prolonged antibiotic therapy, and secondary adverse sequelae (sequelae is a condition following on as a consequence of a prior condition)). There, so now I have told you. Don't say you weren't warned!

I suppose our bodies are simply not designed to have poo floating about in our bloodstream, so they try to make sure that any infection is killed off before it starts. So, if you have to have a prostate biopsy – take your antibiotics!

So, back to the biopsy in question - mine. I was ushered into a little clinic where a doctor (in this case a very beautiful and extremely pleasant lady, I would say of Middle Eastern extraction, possibly Egyptian or Jordanian, maybe Iranian or Iraqi) is standing in a white coat. She checked my identity and that I had taken all of the medications as prescribed, then she proceeded to give me yet another antibiotic by injection into the arm.

Following this, she invited me to loosen my hospital gown and lay on the couch with my bum pointing towards her (see what I mean about dignity?). She then inserted a long, thin, smooth, curved tube with a camera on the end up my Jacksie and said she was going to give me an anaesthetic. Thank goodness for that!!

I didn't feel this injection at all, though others I know said it hurt them.

Then she was fiddling about for a minute or two and then suddenly I heard a sharp "Crack" (see the pun there?) and it felt as though someone had pinched me inside, hard, with a pair of pointed pliers! I cried out and she apologised and said she ought to have warned me! Yeah right – it would have been good!!

Altogether, there were eight of these. Usually there are twelve but not always. I can't really say it hurt; it was just uncomfortable. However, friends who have also had this have described it as "excruciating" and the worst thing they have ever had done. That was certainly not my experience – a dental root canal treatment is far, far worse in my experience even with anaesthetic.

Her loveliness asked me if I had had my MRI scan and I said no, and that I didn't even have a date for it. She said "That's no good, wait here". With hindsight this all tells me that the cancer must have appeared to her to be very advanced, but perhaps I am reading too much into it.

Off she went to return just a few minutes later and said, "If you have time to do it now – I have arranged for them to do it straight away". Yes, please – I could have kissed her, but I restrained myself – not least because I didn't want to be arrested and certainly partly because, given what she had just done to me and after seeing my cancerous insides and shoving things up my crack, I did not think it conducive to a suitable atmosphere for anything like that!

MRI scan duly completed after drinking the ½ litre of Barium. Not Great, Not Terrible to coin the now iconic phrase launched into the world in the Sky Miniseries "Chernobyl" following plant Deputy Chief Engineer Anatoly Dyatlov being advised that the ambient radiation level was 3.6 Roentgen (which it probably is inside an MRI scanner for that matter!). If you haven't seen it, "Chernobyl" is a dramatisation of true events chronicling the 1986 nuclear disaster at Chernobyl - where else? It is atmospheric, riveting, haunting, very graphic and very, very well worth watching.

Sadly, we have just lost the very fine actor who played Dyatlov – Paul Ritter, I believe to a brain tumour.

I digress – sorry. So that was my first brush with scans and biopsies.

CHAPTER 4

Worse news and the consequences

So, my appointment with the Oncologist duly rolled around (yes 2 weeks…. you know by now!) and she also had a nurse with her who I now know is a specialist Oncology nurse who is both professional and extremely knowledgeable as well as very pleasant and very helpful. The presence of the nurse presaged further bad news I supposed.

The Oncologist said, "I have looked at your scans (I assume she did this with her eyes open but they were shut while she was telling me about it) and they show the cancer is in the spine at L5, and on your pelvis and left hip as well as in your lymph nodes". She subsequently forgot - and denied that she had told me about the lesion on my left hip, but my wife was there and verifies this. I shall return to the point much later.

She continued, "I also have the result of your biopsy and this is also not good news. Your Gleason score is 8, that is 4+4 and I am afraid it also shows that the cancer is a rare and aggressive sub-type of Prostate Cancer called Ductal Adenocarcinoma".

Gleason score partially explained (she did not tell me this, I looked it up): They take samples (cores) from each side of the prostate gland. They examine these to see how many of the cores are cancerous and what the cancer pattern is. If the cancer is well defined, this makes it easier to treat so your score will be lower and your prognosis better, but if the pattern is not well differentiated then the score will be higher and the prognosis commensurately less good. 8 is a high score with poorly defined cancer and a considerably less good prognosis, probably regarded as incurable. The Gleason score can go as high as 10. Ergo 8 – (4+4) from only 8 cores is not good news by any standard and perhaps explains why the lovely technician cut the biopsy from 12 samples to 8 as she knew the result was not going to be good and that all 12 would be cancerous if she did them, but I cannot be sure of this. She may have deduced this from my PSA score and the size of my enlarged prostate, or she may only ever have been intending to take 8 cores – truthfully, I don't know.

There is a debate in medical circles as to whether or not biopsies should be 8 cores; 10 cores; 12 cores; or even up to 20 cores. This seems to be a matter of dispute but whatever the case, mine was only 8.

I asked the Oncologist how this affected my prognosis if it is aggressive and given the current spread of the tumours. She answered "I think 3-5 years, probably the shorter end of that range but we don't know very much about Ductal Adenocarcinoma as there is not much research into it, so it is a bit of a guess."

She started talking about starting me immediately on chemotherapy, but I said "hold your horses" (well OK, I didn't actually use those words – I hope) I think I said in my calm and measured way something to the effect that I wanted to think about my options before starting on chemo.

She said OK – but to think quickly and call her in a week with a decision. She also wanted me to start on Prostap injections which is also a hormone treatment for the same purpose as Bicalutamide, but it is a 3 monthly injection instead of a daily tablet – and apparently is more effective. I agreed to the Prostap.

At that point, another lovely lady of Middle Eastern extraction (Iranian I believe but if she reads this and she is actually Iraqi, I apologise – no offence intended) came and explained to me that they were running a trial with Prostate Cancer patients to see whether delivering hormone therapy by way of injections or patches was better in terms of effectiveness and impact on the patient. She invited me to join which would involve me having either the injection or the patches to their randomised choice, and in completing blood tests and a questionnaire every three months. I agreed. They decided to put me on the 3 monthly injections, and I received one immediately.

I went away and I did indeed think about the chemo.

I received a shock when I got a letter from the Hospital confirming my diagnosis and at the top it had a description of the care proposed and it simply stated "Palliative". This actually means providing relief of symptoms and pain for people with terminal or life-threatening illnesses. To me, it simply confirmed they had given up on me although on NHS websites they say it does not mean this. Either way, the use of the word conjures up the impression that that is what it means – you're a goner and they intend only to ease your pain while you shuffle off your mortal coil.

My wife and I decided that we now had to tell our children both of whom were married (still are in fact – to the same people) - 28 years old (Son, Alex) and 22 years old (Daughter, Eliza) respectively. I love them dearly and their respective spouses (Emma and Aymeric). so this was the first truly traumatic thing I had to do in this saga. Their reaction tore me apart as they were, all four, utterly distraught.

I was however, definitely not prepared to die without seeing my grandchildren born, if there were to be any, and at least see them start growing up (and I mean not just as a baby).

In short, I simply wasn't prepared to die for this and all the reasons previously mentioned. No way. No. Just - NO! Think of Margaret Thatcher (AKA The Iron Lady) when, at the parliamentary despatch box in October 1990 she told Jacques Delors "NO, NO, NO!" in response to the EU's wish to centralise power in Europe to Brussels. It simply was not going to happen – not on my watch! (Me dying I mean, not the EU thing).

You should know that my job had also come to an end at this time, just to add to the stress at a time when, as a cancer patient, stress is the worst thing you can have. I and another senior Project Manager were shipped out at the same time and the one remaining PM was put in charge of all projects. Hey Ho, that's life. From my perspective it was a bizarre decision as I had recently brought in the largest project the company had ever had, on time, in budget and with a happy client. What more could they want?

Still, that was their decision. It created some big financial troubles for me which impacted on me in various ways to a very significant degree.

Everything you read about surviving cancer tells you that a positive mental attitude to it is key – it is fundamental to any realistic chance of surviving for any length of time.

So, faced with the trauma of my Children's reaction to the news and my new financial predicament, I called Macmillan[3] for the first time, and I have to say – they are magnificent! Truly, <u>MAGNIFICENT!!</u> Their caring attitude, the range and breadth of advice they can offer you on everything from finances to housing to emotional care and even things like arranging for three sessions of reflexology for me as I had started having panic attacks, was outstanding. They were absolutely magnificent.

Macmillan asked me about everything including how I had coped with telling my children and I have to say I wept at this point. I really cried talking to this stranger on the phone but she was amazing and truly sympathetic, empathetic and knowledgeable and soothing to the spirit and mind - truly a real star. Where do they find the calibre of person that can do this?

If you are faced with this scourge of cancer – don't hesitate, call Macmillan. And raise money for them if you can – they need it and deserve it!

I followed their advice to the letter and was amazed at the dramatic results. Honestly, I cannot praise these people enough.

Anyone who knows me, knows that, faced with a serious problem, my first response is to start reading.

I read to understand the nature of the problem, to understand the options, and then to find a solution that offers the best chance of success or at least the one I can best live with.

---

[3] Macmillan Cancer Support – www.macmillan.org.uk

As previously mentioned, I never considered that I was going to die of this. Honestly, looking back, I genuinely never for one moment believed that this would kill me.

The panic attacks were, I think, a response to the loss of my job and the financial implications of that coupled with the stress of seeing my children so distraught and perhaps some concern at what treatment might lie ahead and how hideous that might prove to be. But not the cancer itself, I was simply not afraid of it.

Eliza and Aymeric had booked a villa near Seville for a week's holiday and invited us to go with them. We jumped at the chance. The only problem was that it was hot – in fact very hot – 46 degrees on several days!! This did not help with the panic attacks but the air conditioning (as old as it was) and the swimming pool, were safe havens in this regard! Eliza and Aymeric were lovely to me there – very solicitous.

I had not 100% ruled out Chemo but was definitely not keen on it. I have to admit that I actually was afraid of that!

Nevertheless, I needed to minimise my stress, and to read, and read fast, so I could get to grips with these problems and come up with a way forward that I could live with.

CHAPTER 5

Research

I scoured the internet for anything and everything on the subject of Cancer in general and Prostate Cancer in particular.

Kind people also gave me books to read on various types of treatments and cures, many of them recommended from their own experiences with cancer and I am truly grateful to each and every one of them for their kindness and concern. I read them all and even if I did not follow the advice from some of these books, I still appreciated it and admired their own application of the information that has obviously yielded positive results in their case. If I did not follow the advice, I did not dismiss it for any other reason than that I found a treatment I felt I could live with and justify to myself.

I also knew the case of an elderly gentleman who was a friend of my family when I was around 5 or 6 years old. He was diagnosed with cancer (I don't know what type) and was told he had 6 months to live. He also refused to die and read everything he could. He put himself on a diet that consisted of nothing but carrot juice – literally nothing but carrot juice. He lived for about 8 years more and with a good quality of life as far as I am aware – he always seemed cheerful. I think he died of old age. Positive Mental Attitude in action.

I suppose I am blessed in this regard; I am naturally a positive person and did not have any battles with myself over being positive – I just was.

My Brother in Arms, seriously, if you are not so positive, I suggest you must try to find ways of building your positivity – I believe it to be absolutely critical with cancers of all types and far more powerful than medicine alone. Seek out and make sure you get help with this if you need it.

I should tell you here and now though, that there is a lot of nonsense out there, some truly wacko ideas in amongst them, in fact there is far more nonsense than material that can really help you. Now, I am going to mention some things below but I am not casting aspersions on any particular forms of treatment I mention, I'm just illustrating the range of stuff available to read about cancer and dealing with a diagnosis.

I shall however elaborate concerning my views on some that I regard as truly positive and some that I have actually had.

There are of course the standard treatments that those in cancer treatment via the NHS will know about: Chemotherapy, Radiotherapy, surgery and various drugs and hormones, and some experimental treatments too. If you opt for these, either by choice or because you just feel you have no other options, then keeping positive will still offer you the best possible outcome, and I genuinely wish for you the very best outcome. But read on – there is also a potential cure (yes cure) that will not cost you very much at all – in fact I would go so far as to say that anyone could afford it.

There are dietary treatments and these range from herbal treatments to grapes. Some recommend making your body system so alkaline that cancer cells cannot live in it, some others argue that Cancer is in fact a fungus.

There are also more scientific approaches to it, for example, Proton Beam therapy (a highly focussed beam that destroys localised cancers with minimal or no damage to healthy tissue) Nano-knife technology where they excise tumour tissue to within a few microns, thus killing the cells, Cryosurgery where they freeze and super-heat the tumour cells alternately until they die, Various types and levels of Immuno therapies aimed at making the immune system fight the cancer itself (some used alone and some used alongside Chemo and other standard treatments) and viral therapies where a virus is created that infects and kills cancer cells. There is also HiFu (High Intensity Focussed Ultrasound).

There is good and bad in many of these alternatives but you need to find the one that suits you best and that <u>you</u> believe will offer <u>you</u> the best chance to achieve <u>your</u> desired outcome, be that a cure, longer life than that suggested by your doctors or simply a better quality of life along the way. This is <u>your</u> choice and although it is a choice you would not have wished to have to make, it is your choice and you *must* make it – there is no alternative to making a choice of some kind – even if it is a choice to do nothing and let the cancer take its course. You also need to weigh carefully, the potential side-effects of your choice on yourself and on those who care about you, and whether or not you (and they) are willing or even able to tolerate these.

Some, in fact most, of these treatments are not available on the NHS and are therefore either available only in private clinics and hospitals or, in the case of herbal remedies etc. you will have to find a source of the ingredients required.

At the outset, I was interested in Proton Beam therapy.

You may recall the case that was in the news in Britain and Europe a few years ago, that of young Ashya King. In 2014 he had undergone the treatments recommended by his team of Oncologists in London for a brain tumour called Medullablastoma, but my understanding is that they could not do anything more for him other than radiotherapy which they knew would cause him moderate to severe brain damage. If he survived, he would be deaf and blind at the very least and probably unable to do anything much for himself.

Prepare for a shock: In terms of success of cancer treatment in children, success is measured purely in length of time the patient survives after treatment and takes *no account whatsoever* of the quality of life they are left with!

Ashya's parents found out about proton Beam therapy, a highly focussed form of Radiotherapy that kills the cancer cells without killing much, if any, healthy tissue around them. They wanted to take their little boy to the Czech Republic for this treatment but his doctors here in the UK refused to release him.

Given that the severe impairment or even death of their little boy were the only possible outcomes in the NHS, they took him from the hospital without their doctor's knowledge or permission, and a truly shameful pursuit of the family across Europe ensued, culminating in their arrest and a disgraceful attempt to have him returned to London to force the British team's views and appalling treatments with known catastrophic outcomes on this poor child.

This viciously Machiavellian attempt thankfully failed, as the High Court finally ruled that he could be taken to Prague for treatment and the family managed to get him safely to the clinic in Prague where he was in fact given Proton Beam therapy.

A subsequent report stated that his parents' denial of Chemotherapy to the little boy had reduced his chances of survival by 30%. However, scans done in 2018 apparently showed him to be free of cancer. Who's in denial??

The boy is still alive and well and reportedly attends a normal school although with some reported disabilities. As far as I understand it, he still has his sight and hearing, and although he apparently will not progress as a normal child, he has quality of life. Surely this is far better than what the NHS doctors could offer him and indeed tried to <u>force</u> on him?

The NHS is not always brilliant and I say this despite having received some good, even great, care myself at times, but at other times it fails and fails very badly as in this case. I notice too that the NHS now has Proton Beam machines and is starting (belatedly and very quietly) to offer this form of treatment in some cases. They sometimes get dragged kicking and screaming to the logical – even obvious conclusion – obvious to everyone else that is, but apparently not to them. But more on this later.

My view is that we simply have to get away from this irrational sense that Doctors are gods or that they know everything, and especially that they necessarily know what is best for the patient – whether an adult or a child. As a society, it is imperative that we now accept that with the information superhighway, many people are now so well informed that they can perfectly well make very complex decisions for themselves about their health and that of their children as well as any needed treatment as other recent cases in the news have shown, and that the role of the doctor should be to enable and support that decision-making process, not obstruct it - except in truly exceptional circumstances.

Ashya King's case, in my opinion, was not a case the doctors should ever have obstructed – I believe they were wrong to do so and subsequent events and the outcome to the little boy himself have conclusively proved this to be so - in my opinion (along with the subsequent purchase of Proton Beam machines in the NHS!). In my view the NHS was wrong on every level and ended up being dragged kicking and screaming with its tail between its legs to the use of this new technology that others were already using and almost at the expense of this little boy's life. All they seem to have achieved was delay and possibly, ultimately, more damage to him than was necessary.

But you know, what irks me the most about this situation with this little boy is that it is symptomatic of an attitude in the NHS. I spoke to my Oncologist much later on about my treatment with CIK[4] (I will return to this in context) and asked her what she would do with my experience if I came back from China cured of Cancer. Her answer sums up the malaise in the NHS and it was that she would do nothing with it as it would be only one case and therefore statistically irrelevant whereas, they need "robust evidence".

Admittedly, one Oncologist cannot change the view of the entire NHS, and probably has no forum for this anyway, but they can record and present information and, in my view, should do so every time they hear of, and see irrefutable evidence of, something that works.

If they never look, how will they ever get robust evidence?! It is Proton Beam Therapy all over again – it seems they just don't learn unless they are forced to. Obviously, nobody could expect them to go trumpeting a breakthrough without evidence – but why can't they at least look and listen when some evidence is presented?

Here endeth my rant – for the time being.

---

[4] CIK immunotherapy – Cytokine Induced Killer cell

CHAPTER 6

The search for treatment

So, I found the same clinic in Prague that the King family found and contacted them. They were extremely helpful and asked me to send my scans and reports.

You can get your scans and reports from the NHS – they are in fact your property. They are pretty helpful with this and will assist you to have them in a format you can use – I got them put onto CDs in a format common in the medical profession. You will be asked to sign a disclaimer regarding GDPR but that is fair and reasonable.

I sent these digitally to Prague and was very hopeful, however, my hopes were dashed a few days later when they emailed to explain that I was not a suitable candidate for PBT due to the Metastasis. It would only have worked if the cancer was contained in the prostate gland.

I had not stopped reading however and was discovering more things that seemed like good prospects to me.

Around this time, a very, very good friend of mine contacted me and said she was devastated to hear about my cancer diagnosis. We talked for a long time during which she told me that she had also had cancer. I was stunned at this as I had no idea.

It turned out that she had been diagnosed with cervical cancer many years previously. Initially, she had an operation and they were hopeful that it had been eradicated. But it came back.

A friend of hers (who I also knew) told her that she had herself been a cancer patient with bone cancer (which I also did not know), but that someone had given her a book called "The Grape Cure" by Johanna Brandt. She had followed the Grape Cure and had been cancer free for many years.

My friend also read the book and decided to do it. She has now been cancer free for 20+ years. (Cervical Cancer has an extremely high mortality rate – remember Jade Goody?). But this is a friend of considerable intelligence whom I have known for many years and whose opinions I trust, so when she told me her experience, I believed her and, in any event, she is still alive and well to tell the tale herself.

She gave me a new copy of the book and I read it, and also another book on the subject by Basil Shackleton (I always have to check his name as I always think first of Ernest Shackleton – he of the good ship Endurance (among other good ships) in the Antarctic).

Both Johanna Brandt[5] and Basil Shackleton's[6] books are fascinating and convincing, but more on this later.

Now, in honesty I have to admit that this is one that I would have dismissed as nonsense were it not for the two people who I know and respect, and one of them being a very good family friend. However, given the living evidence of the success of it, I accepted it, read it, and put it to one side to continue to think about.

By this time however, I had read about CIK immunotherapy and liked the science behind it. Essentially, it involves having a small quantity of your blood taken and then the white cells are separated from it.

These are then manipulated to make them attack the cancer cells, following which they are multiplied in the laboratory into the billions.

These cells are then injected into you via an intravenous drip of standard medical grade saline solution.

---

[5] Johanna Brandt – The Grape Cure – ISBN - 9781570672798
[6] Basil Shackleton – Grape Cure Living Testament – Published by ABE Books – ISBN - 9780722502020

CIK stands for Cytokine Induced Killer cell. My understanding of what this science is, is fairly sketchy but is that Cytokines modulate the balance between humoral and cell-based immune responses. Cytokines are important in health and disease, specifically in host immune responses to infection, including inflammation, trauma, sepsis and Cancer, It is this that enables the CIK to seek out, latch onto and kill the Cancer cells – and kill them they do.

The truth is, that the body should, and indeed does, attack cancer cells naturally. However, cancer cells are clever little blighters and can adopt strategies to avoid being detected by your immune system and then they overwhelm the natural killer cells that everybody has. After that, the cancer has more or less free reign to grow – and it does, very often with lethal consequences.

CIK immunotherapy involves having a huge number of these killer cells injected which literally seek out and kill the cancer cells – rather like having your own fleet of hunter killer submarines searching for and destroying the enemy fleet. When the killer cells find a cancer cell, they kill it – every time – with an astonishing 100% success rate. Once battle is joined, there is only ever going to be one winner, the CIK.

Turning my own immune system on the cancer seemed to me to be preferable to many other methods, and indeed the obvious thing to do as it seemed to me that there should be no, or only minimal, adverse side-effects.

So having identified this as a very interesting potential treatment, I set about finding out if it might be suitable for me and, if so, where I could have it done.

At the same time, I was also pursuing Nano-knife and cryosurgery (I did not know about the viral treatments or the HiFu at this time but would certainly have investigated them if I had come across them and have some information on both which I will present later).

So, where to get CIK Immunotherapy? I started trawling the internet, electronically scouring hospitals in the USA as I thought this would offer the best chance of at least finding it, even if I could not afford it.

I eventually found a hospital that was doing CIK and I contacted them and was fortunate enough to be able to speak on the phone to a Professor of Oncology on the team.

She advised me that firstly, they were only working with blood cancers, and secondly, everyone they were giving CIK was ending up in intensive care, due to Cytokine Storms although she did state that nobody had yet died of it.

About this time, I came across the story of a woman who had breast cancer that had spread everywhere and was now in most of her internal organs. She had been told she had a matter of a couple of weeks to live but was offered this experimental treatment – CIK immunotherapy. She jumped at it. A few months later, she was clear of cancer and doing well. I have been unable to pick up on this story for updates since.

What was happening in the USA however, was that they were (not deliberately) inducing Cytokine storms in the patients. I found out that they were injecting some 90 billion cells into each patient, which seemed a huge number to me, but what do I know?

I read more and the conclusion I came to was that the American doctors were definitely on the right path, but were perhaps simply injecting too many cells thus causing the Cytokine Storm. But again, what do I know?

I also came across a therapy called CAR-T Immunotherapy at this time but my research showed that this too was only being used in blood cancers. Nonetheless, I managed to pull up some scientific papers on both to compare. Sadly, this information went far over my head and way beyond my ability to understand, in fact I still do not understand the difference between CIK and CAR-T.

What I do know is that CAR-T therapy is not commonly used on solid tumours. Rather, Leukaemia patients seemed to be the principal beneficiaries of this treatment – but more on this later.

I found CIK in Germany but they advised that the cost would be around £140,000 and I would have to attend two different clinics in Germany (for reasons I did not get to the bottom of). In any event, £140k was so far out of my league that I did not pursue it very far.

Finally, I found CIK at a hospital in the Dongcheng district of Beijing, China, close to Tiananmen square and The Forbidden City. It is the Puhua International Hospital which is in what was formerly part of the grounds of the Temple of Heaven (a Ming & Qing Dynasty site dating back to 1420, of immense beauty and historical and architectural significance in case you may have heard of it).

I contacted them to discuss it but they would not discuss anything without seeing my scans and reports, which seemed fair enough.

It proved to be quite a problem getting the scans and reports to them in a format they could open. In the end, I had them couriered out to Beijing, so after much to-ing and fro-ing they eventually advised that they had them and had put them in front of their Head of Oncology, a Professor Zhao.

I got a reply the next day (allowing for the time difference which is 8 hours in autumn/winter, 7 hours in spring/summer).

They advised that they would recommend Cryosurgery, CIK Immunotherapy and Traditional Chinese Medicine (TCM). They told me they could offer me a place in the hospital and that, including a room for myself and my wife for 17 days) the cost would be in the region of 260,000 Reminbi or Yuan – equivalent to £30,000. They said the cost could rise to as much as 350,000RMB or around £40,000 if I required further treatment that they were not aware of from the scans and reports.

£30,000 - £40,000. This also was a lot of money especially as I was now out of work, but even so, it was not so much that it seemed totally impossible. But how to set about getting it together now that I had lost my job?

I started thinking about what I could sell and other ways I might raise money.

CHAPTER 7

Crowdfunding and my amazing family

Obviously, my family were aware of what I was doing to try to find treatment. I told them about CIK and about the cost of this treatment. Eliza immediately suggested that she set up a Crowd Funding Page on GoFundMe. I didn't know much about Crowd-Funding but she just launched into setting it up.

We drafted some information and she posted it online within a few days. I have provided the main text she used in case you wish to see it but my site is still available to see on GoFundMe (no longer accepting donations). (See Appendix 1)

Thus started the next exciting instalment of my cancer journey.

Initially, money started dribbling in but the family started making donations to "get the ball rolling" as it apparently helps with getting your campaign noticed if you can get it "trending". Then it started to take off. I am still amazed at the amounts given by some close friends, but this was a humbling experience altogether from start to finish.

I was touched by the fact that in many cases, complete strangers would donate and would say that their motivation for doing so was their own experience maybe of cancer or some other life-threatening illness. Sometimes it was that they had themselves been cancer patients, sometimes they had a loved one with it or had lost a loved one to it, sometimes they were just well-wishers.

Many donors were friends and some were old school friends.

Some were even young children of family friends, who were motivated just because they liked me and asked their parents if they could donate their pocket money which was especially humbling and touching.

Some were previous work colleagues. One of these is a truly lovely young lady called Sophie, with whom I used to often listen to Fleetwood Mac in the studio and who, I had often told her, I would adopt given the chance. She picked up the torch and got many others in the firm to donate for me, Even the boss of the firm who had personally made me redundant just a few weeks before made a substantial donation.

Then, my family swung into action in an amazing way I had never anticipated.

They started fund raising for me - doing coffee mornings, sponsored walks, sponsored golf, sponsored massages, sponsored alcohol-free months, car washing, and just talking to people including their clients many of whom also kindly donated.

My wife was, at the time, PA to the Europe Director of a London Pharmaceutical company and her boss was very kind and concerned and also made an extremely generous donation.

Interestingly, my wife was asking amongst her colleagues about this hospital, and one of them not only knew the place, but had lectured there, in that very hospital! He spoke very highly of it, saying that it is a proper hospital of high international standards. This was greatly comforting to me. After all, China is far away, under a regime we do not understand, and you hear many conflicting things about China.

All this fundraising effort culminated in a sponsored bike ride from London to Brighton and all of my family who were young and fit enough to do it (including, impressively, my wife) took part!! Many of my wife's work colleagues sponsored her very generously too! I was in the support team driving with supplies nearby to the riders and when we all arrived safely in Brighton, we had fish and chips together on Brighton Pier. What a fabulous day and what a wonderful experience! What a family!

What it showed to me beyond doubt, is how much my family love me and that was extremely moving. You never really think about that until something like this happens – but that they were willing to go to so much trouble and expense and commit so much of their time for me was a life changing experience. I had also learned that some of my work colleagues had great affection for me which was amazing.

And, I learned that it is not always the size of the donation that makes it touching, but it is often the fact that someone has thought enough of one to be moved to donate at all. I say it again – and I mean it sincerely - it is a very humbling experience.

CHAPTER 8

China – First sights

So began yet another amazing step on this exciting journey.

My wife and I began to make plans to travel to China.

This starts with the process of obtaining a visa. I started looking online to find out how to do it and there were a number of people allegedly acting as Agents, but it seems now that you must apply directly to the Chinese Embassy if you want to get a Visa.

This is not a straightforward process and you should allow plenty of time if you plan to go this route, by which I mean many weeks.

You must make an appointment to go to the Embassy and they give you a date and a time slot. In addition to the fee, you have to have your passport (which you leave with them once they accept your application) along with other forms of identity and proofs of address.

In addition, if you are going for medical treatment, you must have a letter of invitation from the medical institution concerned. This has to have dates on it, which mine did. So, obviously, this put an imperative on us booking flights which seemed to me to be risky in case they refused us visas for some reason. However, we went ahead and booked with BA on a non-stop flight from Heathrow to Peking or PEK as they call it in the airlines business, Beijing to everyone else now, officially – Peking is the ancient name.

The day of our Embassy appointment arrived and we had to queue outside for about 30 minutes before they opened the doors, and then we had our appointment checked and were issued numbered tickets, our bags were also checked before we were allowed right into the Embassy.

So, we took up a position on seats near the counters and waited for our ticket and counter numbers to come up on the board. Eventually, we were called forward to a counter where we were asked for our application forms and if we wanted a single entry or a two-year multiple entry visa (which means you can revisit) but as it happened, I think the single-entry visa was done away with at that time. In any event, we applied for the multiple entry visa (which, curiously, was the same price anyway!!).

They are very thorough in reading the application forms and asked where we would be staying. I told them we would stay in the hospital. They asked if we would stay together in the same room in the hospital, to which I said "yes".

At this point, they asked for a copy of our marriage certificate. Now, this was not mentioned on any of the forms, but as we did not have it with us, they would not process our application any further. That was it – we had to leave and make a new appointment and go through the whole process again. This is why you need to allow plenty of time – in case of an unforeseen problem! Try as I might, there was no talking our way around the requirement for the marriage certificate.

So, we got a certified copy of our marriage certificate that we could leave with them and made a new appointment.

The next time was the same as the first time with all the queueing etc. but to be fair, once at the counter, they did pick up where we left off previously which shortcut the process quite a bit.

They approved the application, took our fees and our passports and copy of the marriage certificate. Actually, paying the fees was a rigmarole too – we had to go downstairs to pay and this involved another very lengthy queue. Eventually we paid and were told that the passports would be ready about a week later. They contacted us to confirm we could collect them and my wife went back again to do so (they will not post them). The queuing process is the same for collecting as well, so allow plenty of time.

The visa is a beautiful stamp in one of the back pages of the passport with a picture of the Great Wall of China on it – very elaborate, and typically Chinese in its intricacy.

Thus ended this part of my cancer journey, and thus began the next phase…..

Healthwise, I still felt well and now I was excited about going to China, a country I had always wanted to visit. My wife, on the other hand, had never wanted to go to China and had always said she never would and that if I wanted to go, I would have to go on my own. I'll tell you how that turned out later.

So, cut to the next phase….. the journey:

On Thursday November 22nd 2018 just 5 months from receiving my diagnosis, my wife and I, (I think I should give her a name, don't you?) Sheena and I got into a taxi to take us the 15-minute journey from our home to Heathrow. Our flight was due to leave at 4pm. It is a 10-hour flight, so we would arrive at 02:00 in the morning UK time but 10.00 in the morning Chinese time.

We were going on a brand-new Boeing Dreamliner which was absolutely fabulous inside, even in economy class where we were.

In-flight entertainment was great and I watched a couple of films, and had plenty to eat and drink. The stewardess asked me what I wanted with my dinner – wine or beer or other drinks – I asked for red wine and was offered a choice of a Malbec or a Shiraz. I chose Malbec and was given two of those 1/3rd litre bottles – fabulous! (Later she offered me another drink and I opted for the Malbec again and got another two bottles! That's 1.2 litres of wine with dinner – I was happy, in every sense.

We slept a little – there were very few passengers on board and in the end, we laid out across the seats to sleep. It was great.

Friday 23rd November

As daylight rose outside, we were flying over Russia, a huge country, and I was following progress on the flight map on the screen on the seat in front of me that you watch movies on. Then we entered Chinese airspace. The country is absolutely vast and we were flying over what seemed barren landscapes for several hours. Then into Peking – and a good landing.

The Dreamliner flies at 40,000ft and one of the benefits of this (apart from the fuel economy) is that they can pressurise the cabin to a level so that you do not get so fatigued. We felt really fine when we got off the plane and stood blinking and staring at our first sight of China.

The airport buildings are huge, I mean really huge and futuristic. No sensibilities about political correctness in China though, there are signs in Chinese for Chinese people and signs in English saying "Foreigners". You must follow the Foreigners signs.

You have to stop on your way at fingerprinting machines and get your landing card marked as approved before you get to the passport control. Once there, they scrutinise your passport carefully. I ventured a "Ni Hao" (meaning "hello"). The officer responded with a nod. When he finished with my passport, I said "Xie Xie" (pronounced Shi Shi – meaning Thank You) He ignored me. Passport control are the same the world over – miserable people!

But here we were, able now to go for our luggage. Once we collected this, and cleared customs, we had about a 15-minute trip on a shuttle train and we arrived at the building at the front of the airport.

We came out and there was a lady standing there with an idiot board (the name of the boards with passenger names on them). She cheerfully said hello to us and immediately signalled to a guy that was with her to take our cases and put them on a trolley. From that moment, we were treated like royalty – nothing was too much trouble.

The drive from the airport is about 45 minutes and afforded us our first proper look at China – or at least, Beijing. I imagine small town and rural China to be something entirely different but we did not see much of that during our stay.

As we moved towards the city, the buildings became taller and more modern, grandiose even. Some of them are truly spectacular and futuristic designs. Here and there, there is a nod to Chinese heritage with the distinctive curved tiled roof design that is so recognisable but these were modern ersatz versions of the design, much as you see on the front of the Chinese food factories and some restaurants in the UK.

The roads are spectacular 8 lane highways and cars drive so close together I was amazed that there are not more accidents. Most of the signs are in Chinese (obviously – this is China after all) but here and there you see one in English which struck me as curious.

I always like to hire a car when abroad and explore for myself, but I resolved there and then on this journey from the airport that that was not going to happen here! I am quite adventurous with driving in other countries, but this was beyond even my, very tolerant, even blasé, risk acceptance level.

As mentioned, one or two signs appear in English, but not so many that you could navigate by them. However, as you approach The Temple of Heaven area or Tiananmen Square, they are signposted in English and not only tourist sites but some districts and other areas are signed in English.

Another little feature is that these highways have a small road running parallel on each side and on these local buses go as well as little scooters with boxes and flatbeds built onto them as well as tiny single person cars. The scooter vehicles are used as little utility trucks and small taxis, and you might see one going along with a little one-person seat box on the back that completely encloses the passenger and so you might see an elderly lady sitting imperiously in the back as if she were an empress, or another flat-bed type laden with gardening tools. Most of these seem ancient but some are very modern. After a while you notice that they are all electric powered, none of them are petrol driven, so they cannot be that old. China is certainly leading the way with this technology.

Despite this carbon-emission saving measure, there is usually a pall of smog hanging over parts of Beijing which you can taste in the air on really bad days. No wonder that probably 40% of Beijing natives wear masks all the time, and that lung disease and other pollution related health consequences are a terrible scourge in the city.

It has taken COVID-19 to make British people wear masks and even then, many are reluctant in their compliance. Think yourselves fortunate that the air in the UK is relatively breathable in most places.

As you move off the huge main highways around Beijing, you move onto smaller, yet still big highways (6 lanes) and the little parallel side roads become too small for buses, but these are still used for the scooters and other very small vehicles like the extremely small cars they have which are both eye-catching and amusing, but a great idea. It is also amusing to see a normal western style scooter going along with a whole family on it, father driving, mother seated behind him and kids perched on handlebars, on the running boards and clinging onto the back. Not a crash helmet in sight!

We were driving along by a river and the area was becoming noticeably more downbeat when we turned off following the Temple of Heaven sign and I remembered that the hospital is very close to this landmark site and so assumed we were getting close. This, I thought, looking at the rapidly declining opulence level, was not a great sign – what would the hospital really be like? Had I made a mistake? I comforted myself with thinking that Sheena's work colleague had lectured there and said it was a very good, modern hospital.

Finally, we turned into a little side street with Chinese flag bunting at the entrance to the street and proceeded past little grocer's shops and little cafes etc. The cafes looked filthy, I mean seriously filthy, as if you might catch Bubonic Plague just from walking past them! There was even general household washing hanging up in the kitchen areas and dirty pots and pans standing by open windows with flies (and who knows what else) crawling over them.

Derelict tenement buildings were on our left – whole streets of them (when I say streets, you could barely navigate them in a car and only single file if you did). The windows were gone and stuff from inside them was strewn along the streets – all kinds of flotsam that you really would not want to go poking about in for fear of disturbing armies of rats and feral cats possibly full of rabies and other dread diseases.

Then we went around a small dog-leg in the street and things looked a little better. There was actually what looked like a very smart restaurant with large dragon dogs either side of the door and smartly uniformed staff. And then we pulled up outside a large waist-high shiny, sliding concertina metal gate with a sentry box beside it and the security guard inside opened the gate to let us in and saluted.

As we drove along a short drive there were very expensive and very modern western cars parked each side (Mercedes, Range Rovers, Maseratis and so on) and when we got to the end and turned left, there was the entrance to the hospital. It looked like the entrance to a 4- or 5-star hotel in any modern city, all marble and glass.

We got out of the vehicle and were ushered inside while our driver brought our cases on a luggage trolley behind us.

Ada, showed us along a couple of very smart and very clean corridors, past signs (in English and Chinese) indicating directions for MRI scans and CT scans and we were ushered along a corridor to a nurse station. Everything was sparklingly clean and very modern. Several smiling nurses were at the station and they took us along another corridor to our room. I held my breath as the door swung open, but was pleased to see a very modern hospital bed complete with multi-function adjustment facilities and multiple electrical sockets to suit plugs from probably every country in the world.

Our cases followed us in.

So did the man I now know as Dr Zhao. The professor mentioned previously and head of Oncology at the hospital. A very nice man with great and genuine humility which is very endearing, but no English whatsoever.

However, he had with him Dr Nelson Dhu, who is a much younger and taller man and with very good English and Dr Yu Tao, a young petite woman who said little at first. Also a couple of nurses and Ada were there. Ada's English is extremely good. Also Crystal Kang arrived to say hello, she is the one I dealt with at the start when I made my first enquiries. She is extremely helpful and responsive and also speaks very good English.

Dr Zhao said hello and introductions all round were conducted by Ada.

CHAPTER 9

Treatment begins

Dr Zhao's first question (translated by Ada) was "do you have any pain?". I said I did not, but he seemed rather unsure if this could be correct so he persisted with the question via the other Doctors and Ada. I assured him I had no pain until he finally seemed satisfied.

Bear in mind, we had literally only arrived 5 minutes before this.

A nurse took my blood pressure (125/86 which is very good for me – I do have high blood pressure normally for which I take medicines) and my temperature – 36.1 degrees. She also took 6 x small vials of blood for tests.

They explained that they wished to start me on Traditional Chinese Medicine straight away and indicated the Pyjamas on the bed and that I should get into bed now.

Dr Zhao said that they would take the blood for the CIK next day, as soon as possible, as there was not much time for the cultivation process. He also said he wanted me to have an ECG.

He also discussed my cancer history in depth with me via Ada and Dr Dhu.

Then a man in blue overalls arrived with a huge water bottle – similar to the ones you get in offices today, but the largest type. This he fitted onto what looked like a water cooler in a tall cupboard which also housed a fridge. Bizarrely, there is no sink in these kitchenettes, but there are cupboards and worktops and there is a microwave.

The water cooler turned out to be more than just a cooler. It also dispensed hot water – in fact truly boiling water, instantly and as much as you want. It was an excellent piece of equipment and one which turned out to be indispensable to us. Sheena had packed a travel kettle, but we never used it, the water cooler/heater was so good.

The pyjamas were mismatched and amusingly poorly fitting, but after they left, I got into them and got into bed as directed. Sheena began unpacking and we started to take in our surroundings.

The room was air-conditioned and had a small kitchenette, two large wardrobes, a desk/dressing table with a mirror and an en-suite bathroom which had a wet-room style shower, a toilet with a heated seat (yes really) and it had a built-in bidet feature! There was also a basin and a large mirror – all very clean and pleasant.

We had windows along to my right from my position in bed and a TV on the wall in front of me. The TV was near-on useless. You could get about 20 Chinese programmes and France 24 in English. France 24, you soon learn, simply recycles stories all day and all night for 24 hours and sometime the next day too. What an appalling station – watch it for 30 minutes and you have seen all it has to offer for at least 24 hours!

Through the windows, we could see a very pretty little traditional Chinese garden, complete with delicate pretty little trees, some water and a bridge and some Chinese statuary and lanterns.

The other side of the garden is a glazed corridor with rooms off it in which the MRI and CT scanners reside and a line of chairs outside with people waiting for their scans from early in the morning until about 7pm.

There was a folding bed in the room too which Sheena soon discovered was uncomfortable, so we got that taken away and she used the sofa-bed instead which was not much better and had clearly seen better days. We should have taken the deluxe room with a second proper bed in it, but Sheena insisted that as it was £600 more for the 17 days, she would make do! To be fair to her, she never complained.

Mid-afternoon, Dr Zhao returned along with Dr Dhu and Dr Yu Tao who, as it turned out, also speaks very good English. They came to talk with me about the Traditional Chinese Medicine (TCM). I had no issues with this and, indeed was quite keen to get started.

Shortly after this another man in a white coat arrived to do the ECG. He hooked me up to a machine on wheels via lots of wires and electro pads. It was very quick, but I never found out what the results of the ECG were.

Ada popped in again to see that we were OK. I asked if it was OK for us to leave the hospital for sightseeing which seemed to surprise her a bit. I am not sure if they expected me to be much more ill than I was, but I could walk about well enough although I got tired fairly easily and was noticeably slower than I used to be but was genuinely not in any pain.

Ada went off and asked about this – presumably asking Dr Zhao. She returned and said that when treatments were not scheduled, we could come and go as we pleased, but we had to sign out and back in for security reasons. Ada's English is first class.

I asked her how we could get to Tiananmen Square and the Forbidden City. She gave us quite a lot of information and arranged a taxi for us.

We were pretty tired by early evening so after a small repast from the stuff we had brought with us, we were ready to turn in. A nurse came and took my temperature again 36.5 degrees.

Saturday 24 November

In the morning, the first thing that happened was a cleaner arrived to clean the room at about 06:45. This was a bit of a superficial clean, what my Mum would have called "A lick and a spit" but the room was impeccably clean to start with. Nevertheless, she came every morning – 7 days a week.

Shortly after this, a little troupe of nurses we had met already arrived with a trolley, on which was a selection of instruments and a bag of clear fluid containing my Traditional Chinese Medicine.

At this stage, they spoke no English but indicated to me by signs that they had to take my blood pressure and temperature and then set up a drip for me. They very efficiently, and quickly carried out the first two tasks and then opened a pack with a canula in it, cleaned the back of my hand with a medical wipe and inserted the needle. They connected the drip and set it up on hooks that we hanging down from the ceiling. My treatment was under way! I was excited, elated even.

I discovered that the blood pressure and temperature routine take place a number of times each day and they also, very solicitously and with touching reverence, enquire at least once each day as to whether or not "you do poo poo today?".

After they left, Sheena made breakfast, some granola followed by scrambled egg. All very good indeed. I have put a list of what we took with us at the back of the book so that you can get it for yourselves if you choose to go the same route as me. I strongly recommend you do as the supermarkets are distant, and would be a challenge if you are relying on them for basics, particularly if you would want western foods as they are generally very expensive unless they are made in China under a licence agreement. Anyway, Sheena's breakfast tasted very good indeed and was quick and easy to prepare.

Sheena had downloaded an app onto her phone before we left England that translates Chinese to English – this is brilliant and if you go, I would say is a must have.

She used it on the label on the drip bag and we discovered that the fluid contained Ginseng (we were familiar with this), Astragalus Mebranacus (no idea what this is) and Kushenin (also not a clue) – more on this later. She got out her iPad and had to go to get a WiFi password from the nurses. The WiFi was very good but there was not a great deal of helpful information on Astragalus Membranacus and Kushenin.

So, I settled down to await completion of the drip which was about an hour and a quarter.

During this time, Ada returned and explained that she had booked our taxi and that it would be waiting outside for us shortly after my TCM drip finished.

My drip finished, the nurses returned and removed the drip but said the canula must remain in my hand. This, I thought, was a bit of a problem – what if I knocked it and broke it? So I asked for a bandage to be put around it which they did without any issues.

The nurses returned ready to take the blood for the CIK. This, my Brother in Arms, was a rigmarole, but I guess it is important that it is done right first time. They certainly made sure of that.

Several of them (four or five) trooped in with a trolley with all sorts of gear on it. They took my temperature and blood pressure first (again, yes) and then got this sterile kit out which was very elaborate.

They laid out what looked like a large sheet with a slit in it on the bed and with sterile gloves on, pulled my arm through the slit so that it was fully laying on this sterile sheet. I touched the sheet to smooth it out in one place which evoked loud cries in Chinese that very clearly meant "DON'T TOUCH THAT!!!" I didn't do it again!

So, they got everything set up and a nurse was designated to do the deed. I think she was a trainee as the senior nurse was watching her like a hawk. She cleaned a large patch of my arm with surgical wipes and then this yellow fluid applied with large cotton buds so my arm was quite yellow all around the target site by the time they were ready to start.

Said Junior nurse approached with this largish syringe the cylindrical body of which was, I estimate about 10cm long and 2.5cm in diameter. So, she put a rubber strap around my arm and pulled it tight and indicated that I should make a fist so that some veins showed up. She selected one in the middle of my inside forearm which the senior nurse approved, and inserted the needle. She then loosened the strap and told me to relax my hand and started drawing the blood. It was a process that took perhaps 2-3 minutes until she had filled the syringe (Tony Hancock and the Blood Donor sketch was playing through my mind "that's half an armful!"). This was not a painful process in the slightest.

When she had finished, the syringe (minus needle) was placed in a sterile polythene bag and sealed, the whole setup was broken down and they all disappeared with a cheery wave and "you're welcome" in English, in response to my thanks.

I got dressed and we walked to the nurse station and said we wanted to go out, so they got us to sign out and we left.

The taxi was waiting as Ada had said it would be.

Now, I have to say that, given the fact that we had to provide a letter of invitation for medical treatment to get our visas and that they were very keen to know when and where we would be (at the Embassy in London that is), Sheena and I thought that we would be restricted as to when and where we could go, and that we would probably be followed if we were allowed to leave the hospital at all.

This proved to be incorrect. We were not under any restrictions and nobody paid any attention to us. Well, that is not strictly true actually but nobody official took much notice of us.

CHAPTER 10

Tiananmen Square and Forbidden City

The taxi moved off and down to the main road, turning West onto the highway. Before long, we arrived at what was obviously Tiananmen Square and we paid the driver and got out. This place is instantly recognisable. You will recall it became famous during the Student Revolt April – June 1989 when those dramatic images of a student standing in front of a tank were beamed all around the world.

The square itself is closed off by movable barriers and you must enter by a guard post. Here, there was an extremely smart guard standing in a green greatcoat and with a military hat on. Sheena was unwise enough to take a picture of him which elicited some shouting at her in Chinese which clearly meant something along the lines of "It is forbidden to take photographs of a soldier of the Chinese People's Army – if you do it again, I will arrest you and you can expect a heavy fine or prison sentence!". That was my guess at what he said anyway. Interestingly, he did not make her delete the picture.

We found a little shop selling sweets and ventured in. Actually, it was a big shop and appeared to sell nothing but sweets. The only problem is we recognised nothing in the entire shop. Very few of the sweets have pictures of the sweets on the wrappers, and even when they do, some of them are ambiguous.

Anyway, we bought a few sweets, mostly those that appeared to have cherries or other recognisable fruits on them. Some were delicious, like fruit jellies, others were disgusting and tasted like some sort of bland meat flavoured chewing paste! Mostly they were OK, rather than great, but it was fun trying them.

So we moved on into Tiananmen Square. By Chinese standards, we are both quite tall and Sheena is quite striking to look at, especially from a Chinese perspective with her blonde hair and blue eyes and so many of them stared at us and at her in particular. Men and women stared. It was quite amusing really as they would often stare when going past us on one of the little scooters. They would stare quite openly, though it was curiosity rather than rudeness, and several almost crashed as they were going past us not concentrating on where they were going! It was absolutely hilarious!

So, we made our way through Tiananmen Square, past the very impressive Great Hall of the People, and the Chinese National Museum towards the Forbidden City at the top of the square.

What I did not know was that Mao Tse Tung's body is contained in a crystal coffin in a mausoleum at the gate to the Forbidden City for all to see. We did not go to see it. A Chinese dictator is not high on my bucket list of people to meet, even if he is dead.

By the way, officially, the Chinese People still Love and revere "Our Beloved Leader" Chairman Mao. But I got one very educated person, who shall remain nameless for their own security, talking on the subject. I asked if the people really still love Chairman Mao. The response "Of Course – we love and venerate him". A few moments later this person returned and said in a very quiet aside for my ears only, something *completely* opposite.

Close to the gate, a man approached us and asked if we were going into the City. We said we were and he offered to help. Now, I have been around enough to know that people offering their services to unsuspecting tourists like this can be a nuisance and it can sometimes be dangerous, especially in a place where you do not know the customs.

But this guy seemed genuine, and in any event, there were hundreds of people around everywhere. He told us he was a teacher and wanted to show us his work. He took us to the ticket barrier and explained which ticket we needed. He got in for free. He explained that he works in the place so he does not pay to go in.

He took us first to see the place where he works which looked like an artist's studio with examples of calligraphy on all the walls and he wrote our name in Chinese writing in a scroll in large characters. It is very beautiful and we still have it.

He explained that he runs a school, but I was not entirely sure what sort of school this is. I think it is a school teaching underprivileged children ancient Chinese calligraphy. He seemed very proud of what he was doing. He did ask for a donation, and we gave him about £20, which he was pleased with. Were we conned? I don't know, but if we were it was at least very pleasant! He showed us where to go from his studio, told us of a few things to look out for and left us to our own devices.

The Forbidden City is an extraordinary place. It is an absolutely awesome place.

Ming & Qing Dynasties both used and developed this city.

It is huge – I mean truly vast. It is genuinely a city, and if you visit you must allow a day to do so and, even then you will not see even close to everything.

The only thing is that most of the buildings are empty – ironically much of the stuff that was there was destroyed in the cultural revolution under Mao Tse Tung who was both a dictator and a vandal and western estimates say that possibly as many as 20 million Chinese people died (were murdered) in the cultural revolution.

The Red Guard were tasked with destroying "The Four Olds" which essentially meant anything to do with China's traditions and culture which were deemed to be holding China back in the modern world. This reign of terror went on from 1966 – 1976 during which two thirds of historically important sites in Beijing alone were completely destroyed, along with literature and untold priceless Ming and Qing dynasty artefacts.

This, of course, is not in Chinese history books.

Thankfully, The Forbidden City escaped total destruction and has been undergoing restoration for many years.

As you enter, you come into a huge courtyard with no trees. The Forbidden City is one of China's largest and most important heritage sites and was home to no less than 24 Emperors. There are more 980 buildings and almost 9000 rooms. It is in total 720,000 square metres and is therefore almost three times the size of the Kremlin in Moscow.

After the Ming Dynasty, 10 Qing Dynasty Emperors ruled from here up to and including the famous "Last Emperor" the one who was forced to abdicate in 1912.

Building began in 1406 and was completed in 1420. This building frenzy spanned a mere 14-year period but saw the construction of truly astonishingly beautiful buildings.

There are 90 Palace buildings complete with courtyards. It also houses an amazing museum with the world's largest collection of ancient Chinese artefacts from the Ming and Qing Dynasties.

The architecture is stunning with most of the buildings being made of wood with extraordinary levels of detail and complexity especially in the roof construction. The tiles on the rooves are ceramic of truly awesome designs complete with a little procession of graduated ceramic "Auspicious animals" on each corner. Bear in mind that this was all done some 600 years ago when Henry VI was on the throne of England– it is breath-taking and humbling to think that this civilisation was so far advanced so long before our own.

One interesting little factoid – the rooves of the buildings are designed so steep and the ridge tiles too wide for a bird to grip onto, and they are so shiny that birds cannot land on them to foul them! Clever, the Chinese!

Why is it called the Forbidden City? Because common people were forbidden to enter possibly on pain of death, but certainly as a minimum, a beating with rods.

If you go to Beijing – the Forbidden City is truly unmissable – it is only about 6km from the hospital so you simply must make every possible effort to go – no matter how sick you are! Trust me, it is a magical place.

Sunday 25 November

As our bodies were still adjusting to the time difference, we awoke very early – 2am, but were able to sleep again until 07:00.

The routine of cleaner, followed by TCM drip followed by blood pressure, temperature and Poo inquiry followed shortly after the drip was set up.

Nothing else was due to happen that day, so after the TCM drip was completed, we left the hospital, walking East.

After a short while, we arrived at large entrance concourse to something obviously very special. It turned out to be The Temple of Heaven. We wandered up to the ticket barriers and checked out the price of entrance. It was very cheap, so we decided to go in there and then.

This is also a staggeringly beautiful place of Ming Dynasty origin in the 1400s. The same intricate architecture as The Forbidden City and again, building after building all apparently with different purposes. It is a huge area with residences for not only the Emperor and his primary and secondary wives, but also for high-ranking military advisors and political advisors and, no doubt, a large retinue of staff. You feel about as far from home as it is possible to feel in this place. You can't help but imagine the Emperor and his entourage of wives (with their tiny feet as a result of binding), courtiers and priests as well as high-ranking military men as they moved around from building to building and from area to area to carry out their official functions and, no doubt, to enjoy themselves.

Architecturally it is wonderous.

The roof structure on the buildings again is breathtakingly intricate and beautiful with layer upon layer of highly decorated red lacquered beams with intricate designs on them. The beams are built with incredible attention to details and accuracy to create the distinctive curved roof. On top of this are the astonishingly beautiful ceramic tiles which are intensely coloured and the ends of them are finished with roundels with dragon designs, and the ridge has dragon body tiles along it culminating at each end in a dragon head and then down the curves are yet more ridge tiles curved to the radius of the roof and towards the ends are the ubiquitous auspicious creatures, the number and size of which are determined according to the importance of the building and/or its residents.

We got a bit peckish and I bought a pork sausage on a stick. It was delicious. Sheena had some pastries which were also very nice.

At the centre of the complex is the main Temple structure. Everywhere you look is wonder upon wonder of architectural and creative genius in woodworking and ceramics and silk weaving etc. which, when you consider how people lived in Europe 600 years ago puts into perspective just how advanced this ancient civilisation really was.

I was entranced by this place and then, as we left through another entrance (which we discovered was much closer to the Hospital which is actually in the grounds of what was originally part of the Temple of Heaven) you walk along a fragrant tree lined avenue which is both cooling and restful. We noticed Magpies here. which are different to the ones in Britain, but are still definitely Magpies. We also saw other birds here which I cannot identify definitely, but I think they were Eurasian Jays.

The weather was sunny and warm. All in all, it was a lovely day. Isn't that a bizarre thing to say? Here I am, a stage 4 metastatic Cancer patient, ostensibly under a death sentence, undergoing treatment, and yet having truly lovely days out sightseeing in Beijing!!

There are some artefacts to be seen, but mostly this is gardens which are very restful with plants selected for their fragrance and delicate beauty.

Our bodies were still catching up with the time difference and so we had a restful evening in the hospital reading and relaxing.

As the hospital does not provide food, we stopped and bought some very delicious looking cakes and some western-looking bread. The crust of the bread was as hard as iron, but it was a nice flavour, and the cakes were quite nice – lots of what tasted like dates in them.

When we got back to the hospital, I was walking around in jeans and a shirt, but I was told, very firmly, that I had to get back into bed, that I could leave the hospital when I chose but, whilst in the hospital, I had to behave like a patient. They have a very strong sense of propriety!

Sheena had taken lots of provisions because we knew before we left London that the hospital does not provide food. So we had dried egg (which turned out to be delicious) milk powder (also delicious – tasted genuinely like blue top milk), porridge, dried soups, dried vegetables and other stuff. Her foresight made it a very comfortable experience to self-cater in this hospital. See the back of this book for a complete list of suggested provisions to take that are lightweight, easy to pack and are not likely to fall foul of the strict importation rules.

Around 7pm, the dayshift nurses came in and said goodnight, waving and smiling. About 20 minutes later, the nightshift nurses came and said "Hello" – in Chinese and also waved and smiled. These people are delightful – smiley and friendly.

Blood Pressure and temperature routine duly performed by the nightshift, we settled down to read our books but were quite tired after our journey and the day so we soon turned off the lights to sleep.

In the night, they come in and check on you several times, I supposed in case you had 'popped your clogs' and they needed to get you on the wagon in the morning when they came round ringing the bell and shouting "Bring out yer dead!" (that was a joke).

They didn't check pulse or blood pressure or temperature, simply walked in, looked at you and left – 8 times out of ten leaving the door cracked open which was irritating as it let light in, which shone directly at me! So I had to get up to shut it.

Nobody died while we were there – at least not as far as I am aware. I suppose it happens, it is a hospital after all and, by definition, the inmates are all sick. In fact given that it is an international hospital and that very few patients are Chinese (most Chinese cannot afford it) these are people who travel from far away at great expense to get treatment here, so they must be pretty sick like me, and it therefore follows that it must happen that one 'falls off the perch' every now and then.

Take my own case, a death sentence from the NHS had brought me to Beijing. Notwithstanding the cost, I was still not sure if they would be able to cure me or even buy me much time, even though what I had read about CIK gave me great hope. That was not even really the point – I simply had to try. If it worked – great. If not, then I had lost nothing and seen some wonderful things before I clocked off.

CHAPTER 11

Pattern of hospital life emerges

Monday 26 November

Slept well overall, but still awoke at 02:00. Had a cup of tea, but managed to go back to sleep and was awoken by the cleaner coming in at 07:00.

At 7:30 in came a couple of nurses with the trolley and drip. They checked Blood pressure, temperature and pulse and made Poo enquiry before setting up the drip again. As they left, I said thank you and they responded with a smile and "you're welcome" in English with a Chinese accent which made it sound special.

Sheena got out Granola and fruit for breakfast while I was on the drip. It tasted good. Coffee to follow and that was done. Very nice.

Dr Zhao and his entourage came in and we discussed how things were going but not much to report at this stage.

They removed the spent drip and then we were free for the day.

We were introduced to Cathy as our new Coordinator as Ada was having a holiday. Cathy is very knowledgeable and extremely helpful. Her English is near faultless. (They all take western names for themselves when they are children. These are decided by the child themselves and mostly, they like quaint English names. One of my Doctors, as mentioned, is called Nelson – he was good fun).

Cathy was something else! As we got to know her, we became very fond of her. Nothing was too much trouble for her. She loves Hip Hop dancing and has a great sense of fun as well as huge knowledge of Beijing which proved very useful to us.

We wanted to visit a supermarket to get some extra stuff and Cathy arranged a taxi to take us to a Carrefour (French supermarket chain) in Central Beijing.

If you buy Chinese stuff or local produce, it is very cheap. But if you want anything western it is very expensive. Wine for example – nasty French plonk will set you back at least £25 a bottle! You can get western beers too, Budweiser, Coors and so on, but the Chinese beers are very cheap and very drinkable too, so no need to spend a lot on that.

In the deli section, there are all kinds of things that look like meat, but that I would not buy for fear of not knowing what they are. Even snakes are sold here, from big ones to little ones, many varieties. Again, not for me!

We did buy some cooked duck but to be honest, there was precious little meat on it – it was almost all bones, so we didn't do that again!

Fresh fruit is very good there and we stocked up on a few things including a couple of tins of what appeared to be recognisable as luncheon meat for sandwiches for our days out. One tin was good, the other was truly disgusting, so be careful!! China is a very long way from home and things are not always what you might think!

We also spoke to Cathy about having Peking Duck. I figured that you cannot get more authentic Peking Duck than in Peking so we had to try it.

Cathy recommended the oldest and best Peking Duck restaurant in Beijing which is identifiable by having two large yellow ducks outside the door, one either side.

She again arranged a taxi for us. It was a beautiful day 25 degrees plus and bright sunshine again.

The restaurant is indeed easily identifiable by said two large yellow ducks one either side of the door. We went into this beautifully decorated restaurant which I remember as predominantly yellow with red trimmings. The staff were impeccably dressed in yellow silk garments in typical Chinese style.

We were shown to a table and sat while the table was set up for us with various items and then we were passed the menu. The first thing I noticed was that the menu was all in Chinese with no translations and no pictures. There were no pictures on the walls – this was clearly a classy restaurant, not a cafeteria.

I called a waitress over, or rather indicated that I would like to talk with her. She had no English. In fact, what soon became clear was that not one of the staff speak any English whatsoever – not a word.

After a few minutes, the Maitre'd came over and very calmly took charge. She was brilliant. She recommended (by pointing at what others were having) the Peking Duck – which was after all what we had gone there for and I believe was pretty much all they did anyway.

I saw some beer on an adjacent table and both the lady and the gentleman were drinking it, so thought it must be OK to have this, so I indicated that that was what we wanted.

When the Duck came, it was a revelation. It came on a trolley with a chef, and the Maitre'd was in attendance talking to him. He first sliced a thin piece of skin off the duck for each of us and put it on our plates. It was crispy and absolutely delicious.

Then, he began shredding the duck meat off the carcase which he did amazingly fast and soon it was completely clean of meat.

The Maitre'd put this in a dish on a little heater on the table and a bamboo basket with a lid on it which contained the pancakes. She then performed a task that I still cannot quite believe I saw. With chopsticks, she took a pancake from the basket, set it on Sheena's plate and then proceeded to put meat and other things on it along with some sauce and then she rolled the pancake up into an absolutely perfect pancake roll and showed Sheena how to eat it. She never touched anything with her fingers – it was truly astonishing how fast and accurately she did this.

She repeated the exercise for me and then bowed so charmingly to us and left.

We continued through our meal, trying as best we could to emulate her skill but with only limited success. Nevertheless, it was a gorgeous meal.

With another drink each, the whole meal came to just 175 Reminbi (Yuan) the equivalent of £20. We had read our tourist guide and had asked Cathy about tipping, but it is not generally done in China, nobody expects it and it may even be offensive in some places.

Getting a taxi back to the hospital was a challenge. It took us nearly half an hour to flag down a taxi but finally, we got one and we showed the driver the card Cathy had given us which is printed with something to the effect "Please take me to Beijing Puhua International Hospital at……" and it gives the address. We got back and were very happy.

Night fell, the day staff trooping in to say goodnight and the night shift trooping in to say hello now became a routine but a welcome one – these nurses are truly lovely, sunny and bright and very good humoured. They make you feel like a celebrity.

We retired to bed to read and settled down for the night.

The routine of the night nurses coming in to check on me also continued as did them leaving the door ajar, to my frustration!

CHAPTER 12

On the scans merry-go-round – again!

Tuesday 27 November

Woke at 7.30am after a good night's sleep. What was now established as a routine began with the cleaner coming in followed by the nurses with the TCM and the routine of Blood pressure etc. Blood pressure a bit high at 142/97 – second reading worse at 151/90. Had breakfast prepared by Sheena, scrambled Eggs and bread. Lovely.

The TCM drip finished and a nurse came to remove it and she removed the canula too. Another nurse entered soon afterwards and inserted a new canula before administering a contrasting solution for the CT scan from a syringe into the canula.

Dr Zhao and team came in and we had a consultation again and he explained what was going to happen via Cathy, Dr Dhu and Dr Yu Tao. I was happy that things were progressing.

I got up and showered – again the shower was cold as I was late into it. The reason, I discovered, is that they have solar heaters on the roof, but in the winter, it doesn't heat enough water for the whole hospital, so you have to be early into the shower if you want it hot. This was the only facility I found during my stay that was less than excellent – apart from the TV already described, which was absolute rubbish.

Still, I was feeling good, marvellous in fact, and a cold shower was simply bracing!

As I emerged from the shower, a nurse came in and told me I had to go for the CT scan. She told me to put PJs and dressing gown back on. I did so and followed her around to the corridor I could see from our room and sat on one of the chairs looking back across at our room. There were some people in the queue that looked very sick indeed.

I was waiting until the person who was already in there came out and then was jumped up the queue to go next which made me feel a little guilty as the very sick looking ones (mostly Chinese) had to continue to wait.

The scanner is a Siemens model similar to the ones in the NHS and it looked brand new. I was loaded onto the now familiar sliding bed and the scan commenced, following the pattern I knew from the UK.

Scan finished and I was led back to my room.

No sooner had I arrived in my room than another nurse arrived and told me I had to go for an MRI scan. Same procedure including jumping the queue but the MRI scanner is in the adjacent room. Scanner again looked almost brand new. I was loaded onto the familiar sliding bed and the scan commenced with the same small tube arrangement as the UK. I shut my eyes and thought of something else.

Scan finished and I was led back to my room.

I had been back around 2-3 minutes when the door opened and the first nurse was back saying I had to go for another CT scan. This seemed somewhat bizarre, but hey ho, I had little option but to comply. I jumped the queue again with some of the same people still waiting as at the first time! I felt worse about that, but what could I do except what I was told?

Scan duly completed and I returned to my room only to have the second nurse walk in to tell me I had to go for another MRI! I asked why, but she shrugged and indicated I should hurry.

Second MRI duly completed and I returned to my room hardly daring to sit down in case I was summoned for a third CT, but no, that was it.

We settled down to wait for a bit to see if anything else were to happen, and it did.

About half an hour or so later, Dr Zhao and team plus Cathy returned.

He announced that the scan results showed the prostate cancer had almost disappeared from the prostate, in fact they could not find it at all! But 2 x tumours in the spine at L5 were still showing clearly and 2 x small tumours in the hips. Professor Zhao said the tumours in the lymph nodes were smaller than in the earlier scans done in England. I asked why this should be.

He said he thought that the hormone therapy was working and, combined with the TCM was having a dramatic effect in shrinking the cancer. He confirmed that my latest PSA score was 1.75.

I asked him what, considering the CIK I was going to have, would he think my new prognosis would be?

He gave a reassuring prognosis of life expectancy which he just said would be well beyond 5 years! He also suggested that I could change to another hormone when Prostap becomes ineffectual. He said there are a number of hormone therapies available.

I felt very happy.

MY EXCITING CANCER JOURNEY

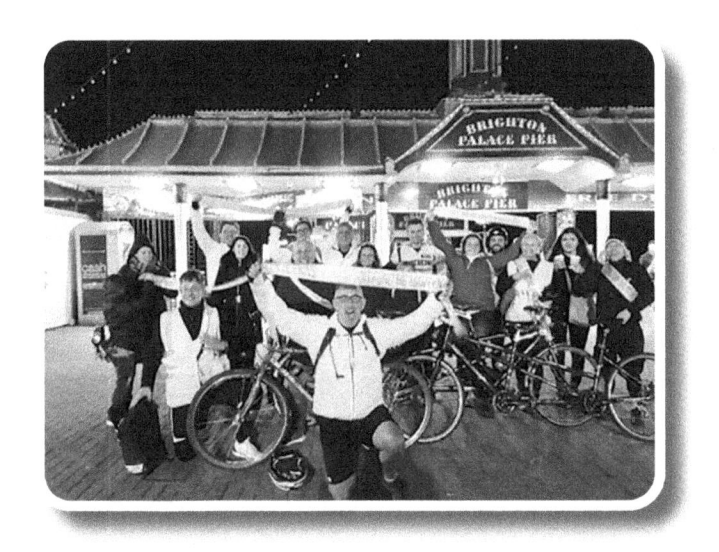

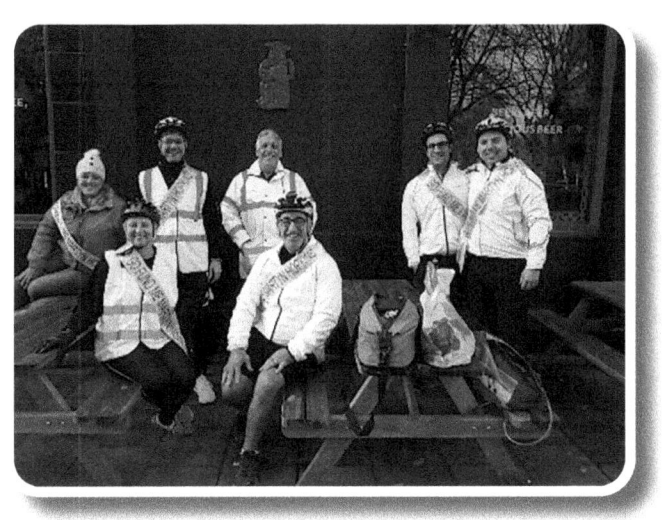

London to Brighton sponsored cycle run

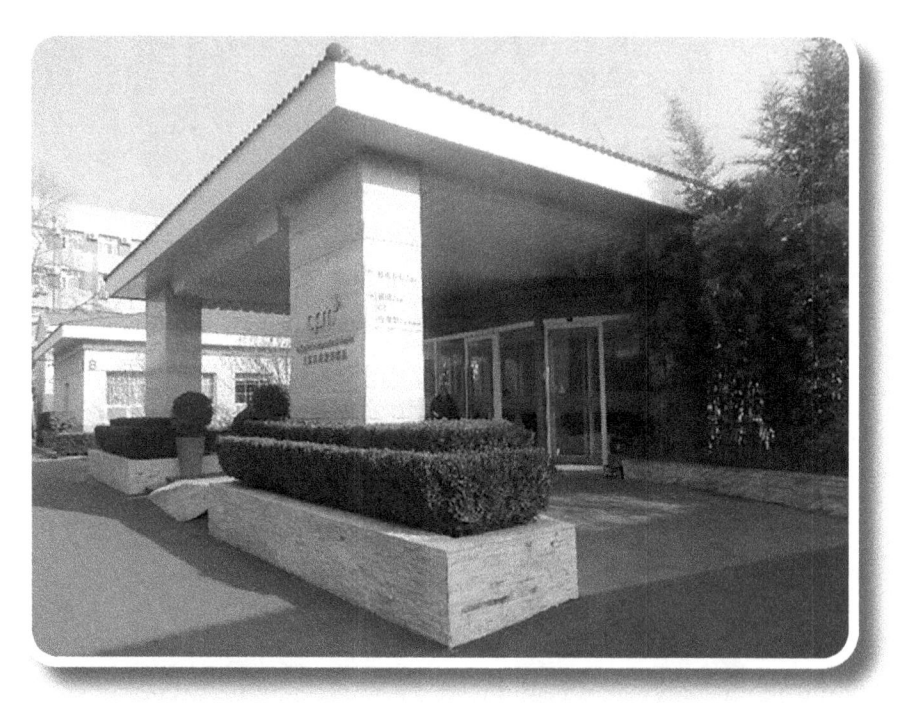

Entrance/Reception Puhua International Hospital, Beijing, China

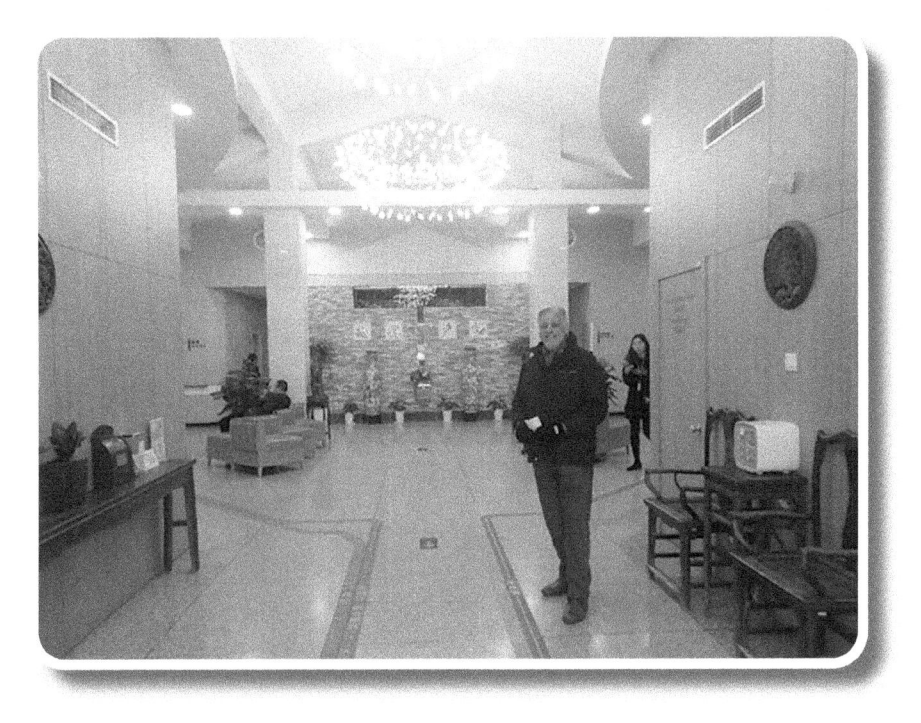

Inside the Beijing Puhua International Hospital

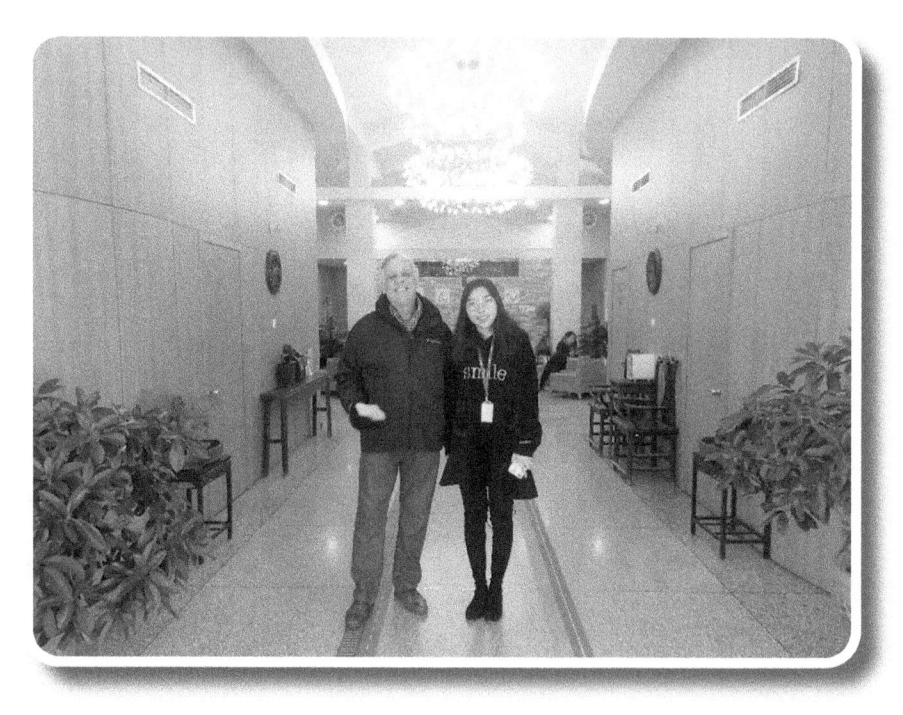

With Crystal Kang – overseas administrator

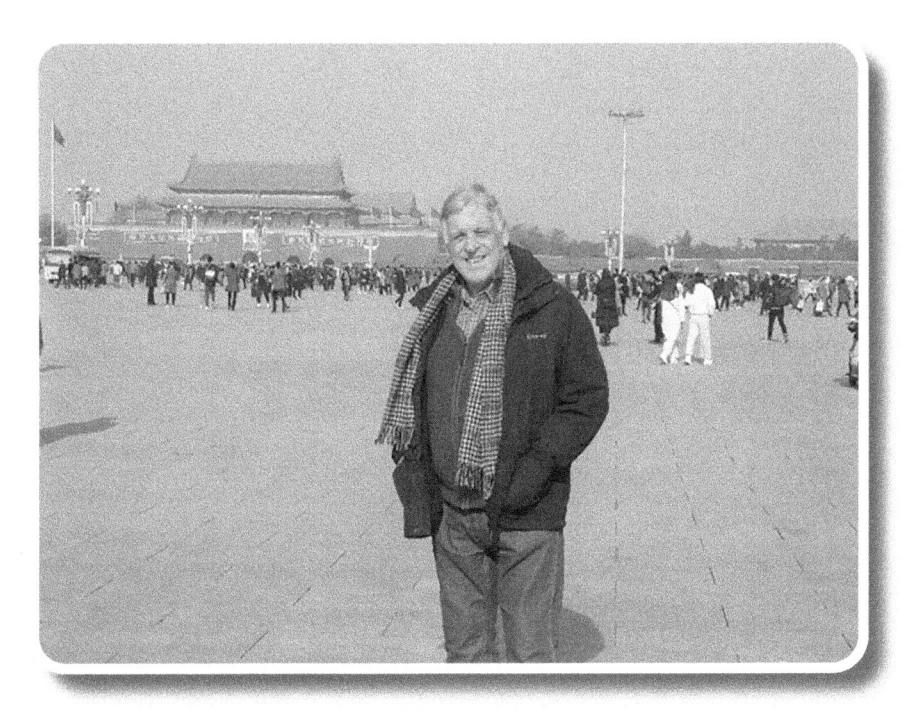

Tiananmen Square, Beijing

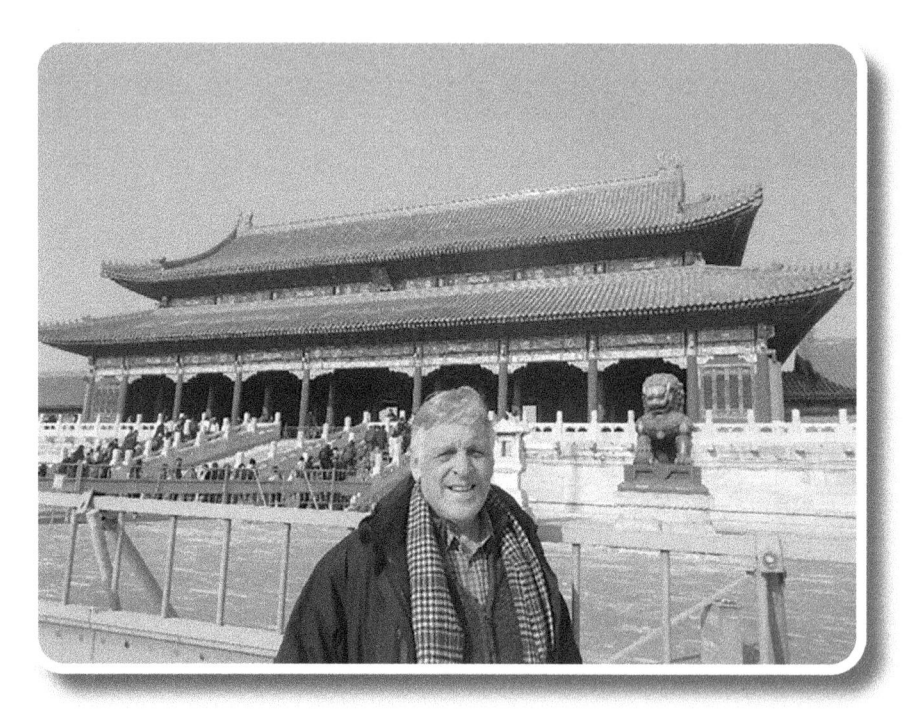

The Forbidden City, Beijing

MY EXCITING CANCER JOURNEY

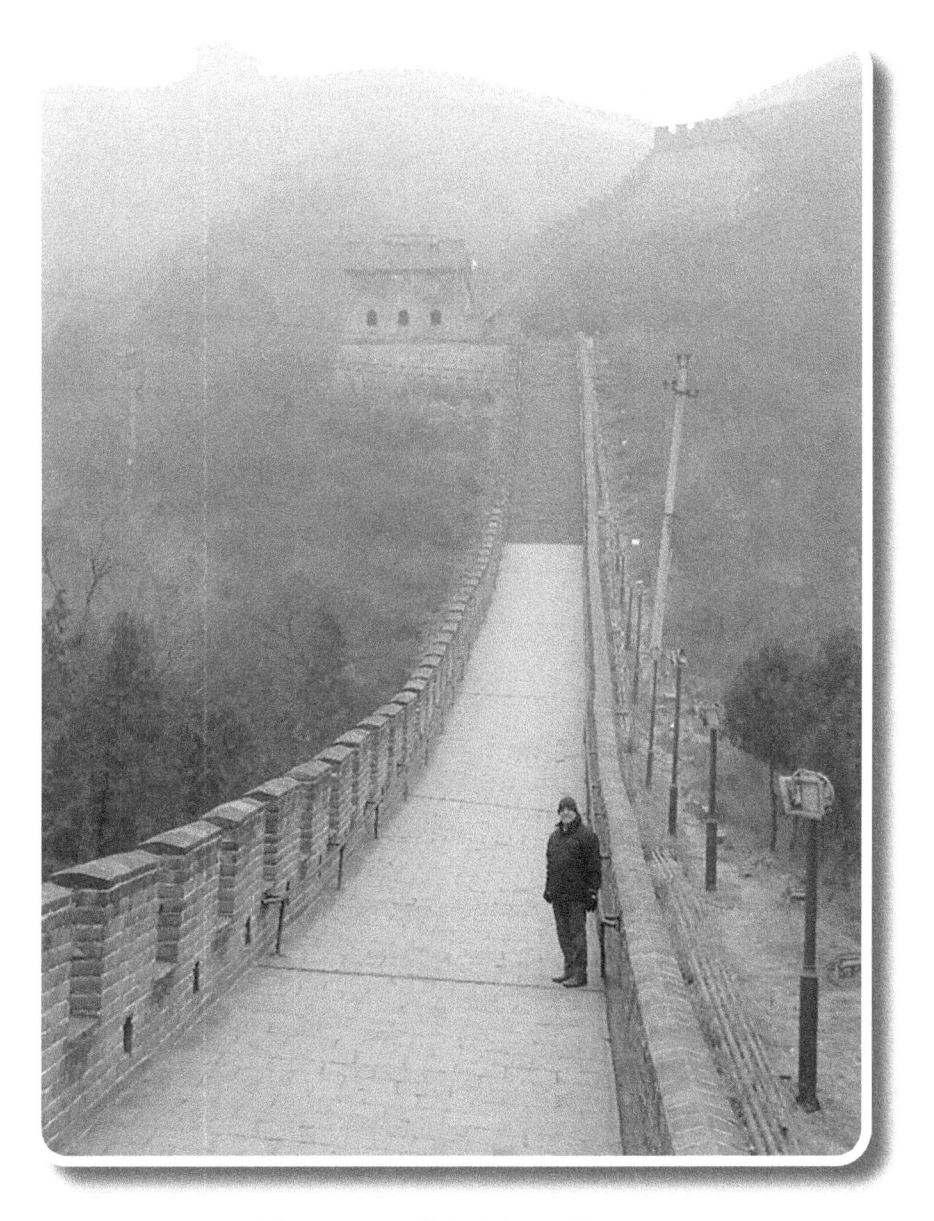

The Great Wall, Badaling, China

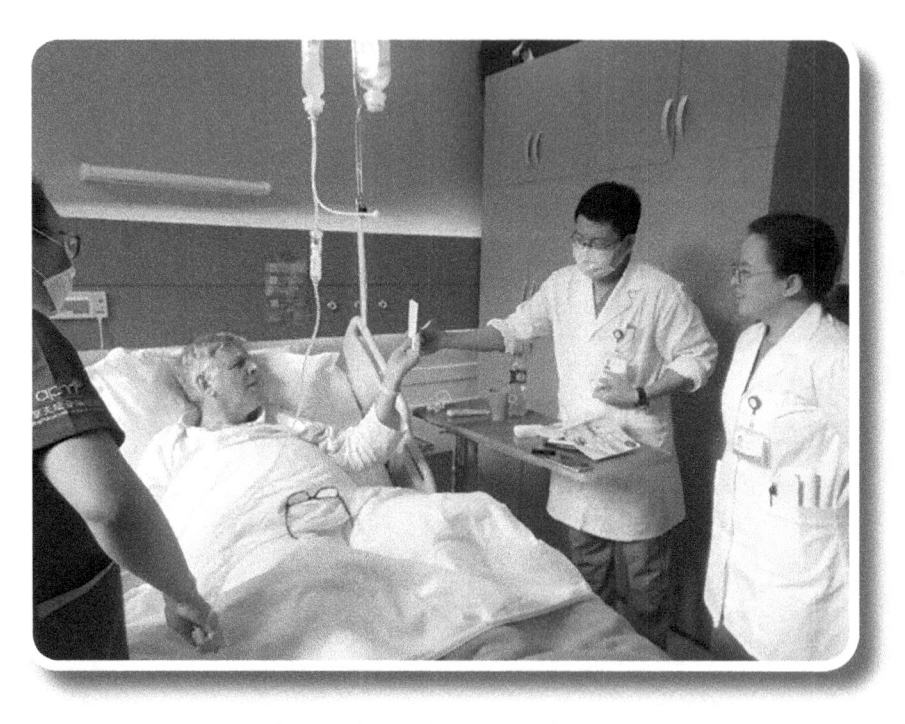

With Dr Dhu and Dr Yu and Nancy
administering the CIK immunotherapy treatment

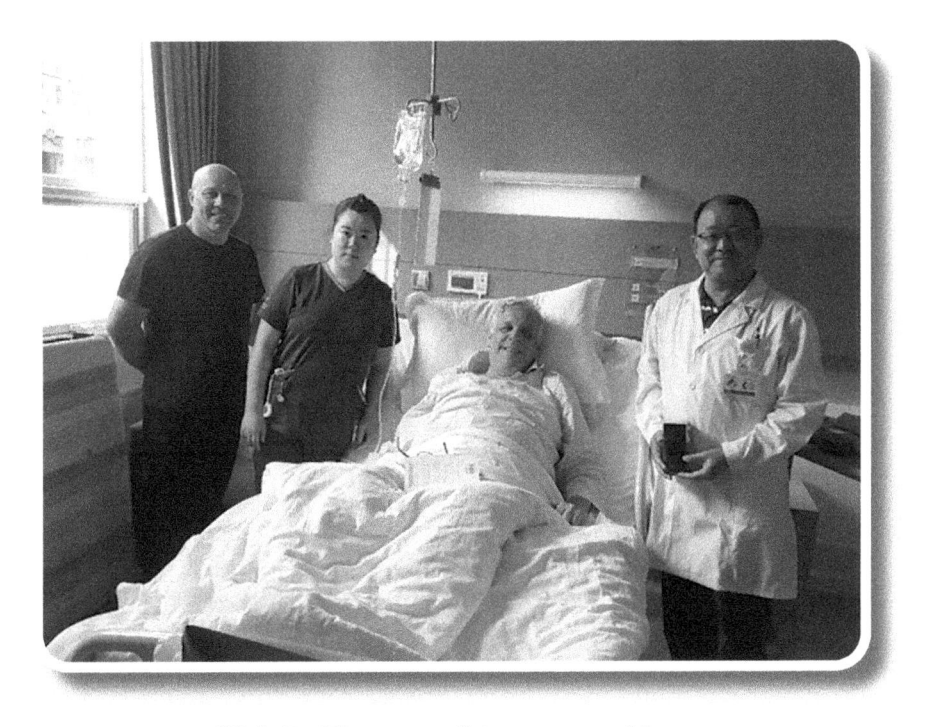

With Dr Zhao, one of the nurses and Ian

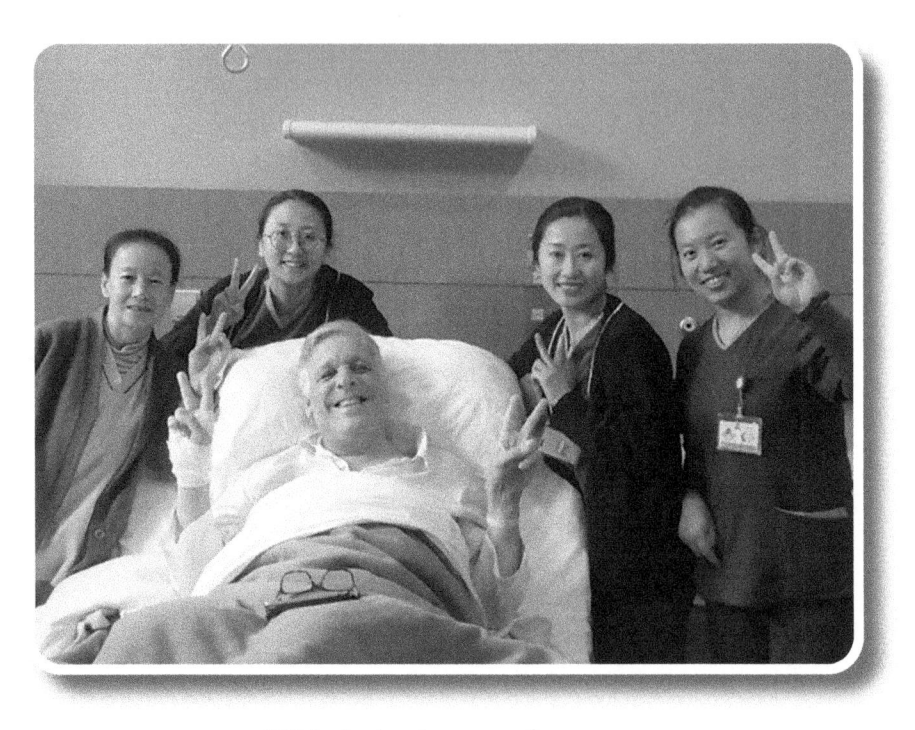

With the lovely team of nurses

MY EXCITING CANCER JOURNEY

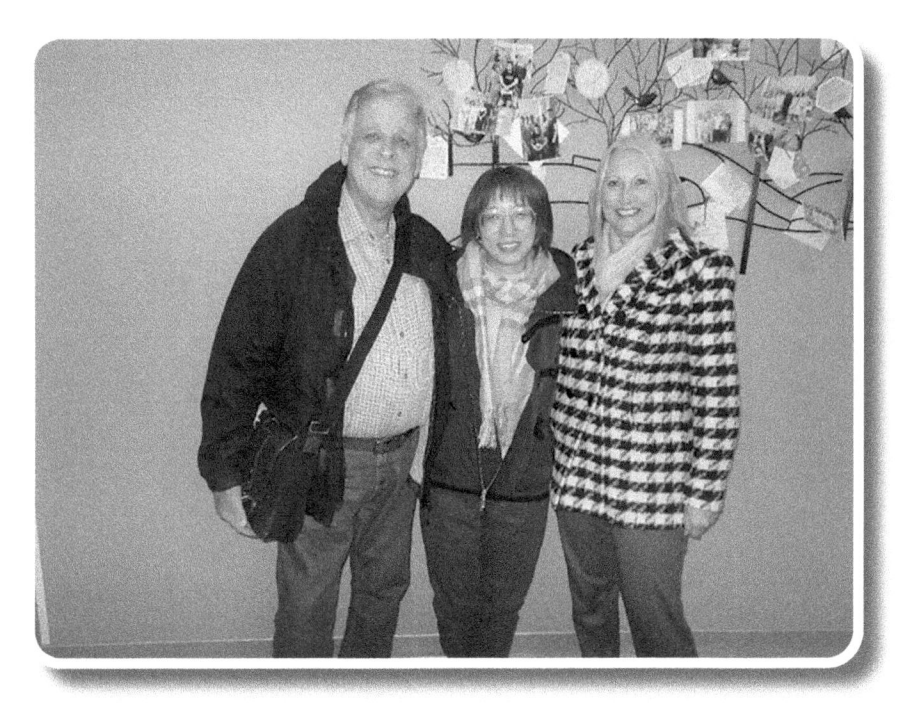

With Cathy Wang and Sheena

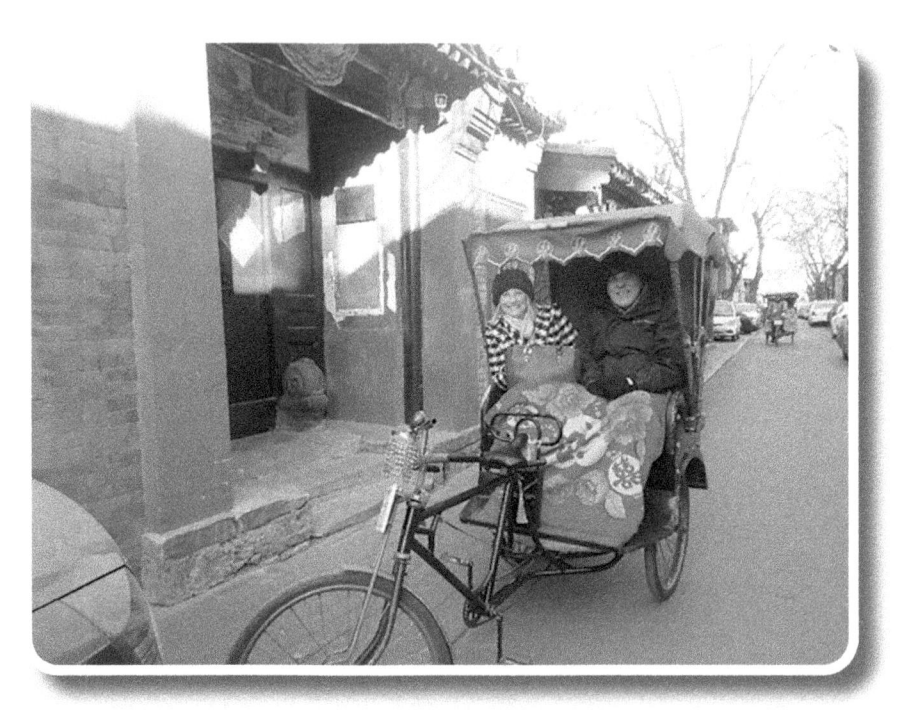

With Sheena in a rickshaw visiting the Hutongs

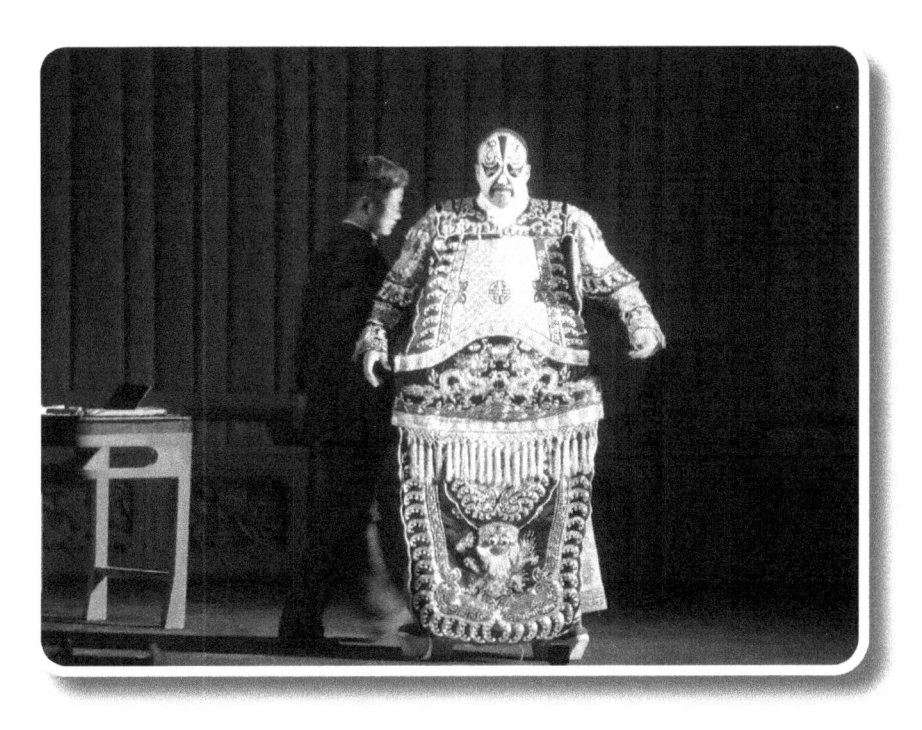

Chinese Opera costume demonstration

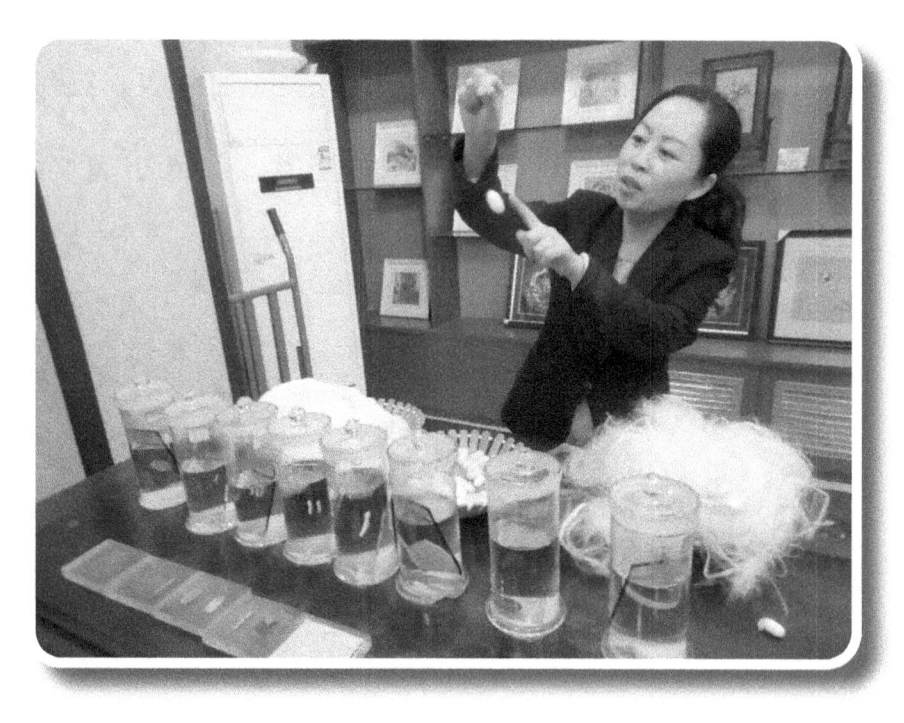

Visit to a silk factory

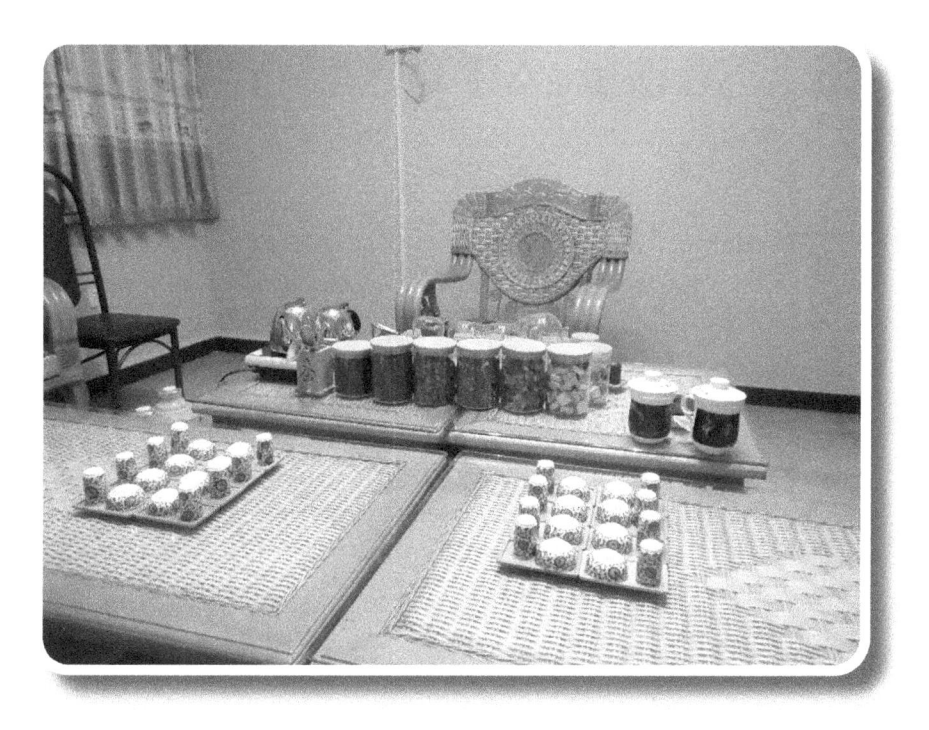

Visit to a Tea House

CHAPTER 13

Silk Street and Western Cakes!

Treatment finished, Sheena and I went for a walk, going on the route past the Temple of Heaven entrance and towards a large flyover that carried the inner ring 8 lane highway.

At the bridge, we turned left and continued walking along by a parade of shops, one selling Trainers and nothing else. They looked very cheap but all the top brands were there and some I had never seen. I wondered if the branded ones were genuine or clones.

Then we saw a bakery which looked amazing. They had western looking cakes so I bought a large cream bun, Sheena had another cake with cream and we bought a couple of French Batons that were absolutely fresh and tasted wonderful!

We walked on much further to a large building with multiple small stores inside it and here we bought silk scarves and ties. We saw the same silk ties that we had seen at a silk factory store, but at a hugely inflated price – about 6 times the price. The store owner was very, very keen on getting a sale, so I started bargaining with her – in English – hers was pretty good. We wanted several ties for the guys in the family and they were very nice, so I started bargaining very hard. I told her that we had been told that they mark up the prices by 10 x times and that I only wanted to pay the base price (which would have been a cruel price to pay). She feigned horror and walked away, but soon came back. She offered a price that was about twice the price in the silk factory so I just laughed and went to walk out of the shop.

She ran after me to the door and brought me back inside as the age-old elaborate dance continued, and then the real negotiation began as she knew that I knew what the price really should be. Eventually we got there to actually just under the factory price, so I knew she really wanted this sale very badly. We bought them and a couple of scarves – but we hardly needed to haggle on these as she gave us the factory price to start with!

A really miserable and grumpy taxi driver took us back to the hospital! I suppose Taxi drivers are the same the world over. It was probably because I did not accept his price but insisted that he use the meter which gives the regulated fare. It was about 20% of what he had asked for. We were learning!!

Back at the hospital, a nurse came in carrying a large polythene folder with a wadge of very large scans in it. These were acetates about 600mm long x 450mm wide (2 feet by 18 inches in old money). I had a look at some of them but couldn't make out too much of significance. I still have these since, despite them being very heavy, I could fit them in my case and wanted my UK Oncologist to see them.

Cathy came in and asked if we were OK and we had a lovely chat with her, she is really delightful and great at her job. We settled down for the evening reading and online with our iPads.

Day nurses came and said goodnight, night nurses came and said hello and the night routine began its now usual pattern.

Wednesday 28 November

Woke at 6:00 today after another good night and the now familiar routine began. It was still very bright and warm outside with clear blue skies.

The nurses set me up with TCM drip again.

Then another two nurses came in and said I needed to have a Prostap injection as the last one in the UK was 3 months prior. They wanted to deliver this into the buttocks or belly but I didn't fancy that so I asked if it could go into my arm. Mistake!

It was painful going in and resulted in a hard and painful lump! This persisted for about a week before it dissipated, so I resolved not to do that again!

Sheena made breakfast using the utterly delicious French bread we had bought the day before. This bakery was now firmly on our list of shops to go to!

The door opened about an hour later while I was still on the drip, and in trouped Dr Zhao, Dr Dhu, Dr Yu, another two doctors I had not met and the senior nurse – and Cathy. Seven of them!

Hmm – something is afoot methought!

Dr Zhao, as always, led the consultation, this time with interpretation by Cathy.

Firstly, he introduced the CIK specialist and the Cryosurgery specialist. The others, we already knew.

A lengthy conversation in Chinese kicked off proceedings which, obviously, I did not understand. At the end of it, Dr Zhao gave a nod to Cathy and she started to tell me that there was some news.

It turned out that the Cryosurgeon's opinion was that the tumours were invisible on the new scans and so he could not carry out the Cryosurgery on the prostate. I was not entirely unhappy about this on two counts: 1) They insert the implements for Cryosurgery the eye-watering way – through the small opening in The Honourable Member for Littlehampton! 2) this was surely great news that the tumour in the Prostate was now so small it could not be seen. Dr Zhao agreed vigorously on this second point.

His opinion was that the hormone treatment started in the UK, combined with the TCM was having a dramatic effect.

I asked if the Cryosurgeon could carry out his surgery on the spinal tumours instead. This resulted in another very lengthy confabulation of about 10 minutes in Chinese which Dr Dhu translated for me.

He said that the Cryosurgeon was not willing to carry out Cryosurgery on the spine as the risk of paralysis would be too high. I asked how high a risk we were talking about and Dr Dhu spoke in Chinese with him before reverting to me with the news – 50/50. I immediately agreed this risk was far too high and that was the end of that.

The Cryosurgeon nevertheless remained with us until the end of the whole consultation.

Dr Zhao then started talking again via Dr Dhu and Cathy chipping in from time to time. Dr Zhao pulled out some scans and showed me these and explained that what he had originally thought were tumours on my L5 vertebra were in fact calcification. He elaborated and said that it was impossible to see if there was still live cancer under the calcification, but that it was good news, although the calcified bone would be more brittle than normal bone, it at least showed the cancer is dying, which is, obviously, the main intention.

He then brought the CIK specialist into the group discussion. However, apart from indicating that the CIK would go ahead as planned, there was not much to add.

There then ensued a discussion about taking further blood for a second cycle of CIK should it prove to be necessary. This was agreed as the culture could be stored for up to two years.

Professor Zhao recommended that I stay on the Bicalutamide and Prostap for the time being and arranged for a quantity of Bicalutamide to be sent to my room as I had not brought any with me.

He enquired as to how I was feeling and, frankly, I was feeling a million dollars. He said the TCM would be doing that and he was very glad that I was not feeling so tired now.

They all left after further general discussion. It was all very pleasant.

Dr Yu Tao returned a few minutes later. She had not said much even though she had been in on each visit of Dr Zhao. But now she chatted with us and we discovered that her English too is excellent. She is a very intelligent and witty lady and we enjoyed chatting with her, the conversation ranging over life in China, places to visit, food and much more. She too is delightful and very great fun. We liked her very much.

We were becoming very fond of these people with whom we were now building a warm relationship.

After this, we had cheese rolls made with the butter and Cheddar we had brought from England in the French bread from the local western style bakery. Delicious!

After this lunch, we went in search of the museum of architecture I had seen on our tourist map of Beijing. On the way, we saw one of the old gates of Beijing which has been restored and preserved. There is a large square leading off from the gate where people fly kites, which is a national pastime. Here and there, were also little groups of old men playing Mah-jong.

The kites were fascinating, some of them were shaped like birds and at a height they are very convincing. Some are box kites even very tiny ones and some are like rollers that spin while the kite is in flight. Some are dragons with long and exotic tails but it is all very colourful and interesting. They fly these on strings that are immensely long and the kites fade off into the far distance. It is an amazing sight.

The Museum of Architecture is a fascinating place, but a fair trek from the Hospital. Anyway, we found it and again, it was inexpensive to get in. We spent a couple of hours going around this place where we learned how they built the immensely complex roof structures in ancient times and much else besides. This is a great place to while away a couple of hours.

Walking back the way we came we were passing what seemed to be a large stadium where it looked as if a football match or some other event was to take place this evening. I was very uncomfortable with the men standing around outside as they eyed us in a rather unpleasant and slightly threatening way. I have to say it was the first, and indeed the only, time I felt at all threatened in Beijing. Nothing untoward happened and we made our way back to the Hospital, but it was not comfortable walking through a crowd of these guys some of whom were obviously talking about us and not, seemingly, in a nice way.

We laughed again at all the funny little vehicles driving around, they really are comical to a western eye! Having said that, they are extremely practical and utilitarian.

CHAPTER 14

Cryosurgery refund

On arrival back at the Hospital, Cathy came to see us.

She said that as I was not having the Cryosurgery, they would refund the payment I had made for it. I was amazed, I had not even had to ask about this. I asked her how much it would be, and she said the accounts department had to fully check it, but she thought about £12,000.

One thing I should tell you about this hospital is that you have to pay before you arrive. However, although this is a profit-making enterprise, they are not primarily money motivated. As an example, when I arrived, the money I had sent from my bank in London had not cleared into their bank, but they began my treatment immediately anyway without any concern – they hadn't even checked if the payment was in until I asked. And, as the matter of them refunding money to me for treatment not undertaken shows, they are very quick to refund when it is necessary. The refund was back in my account in London (it was just over £12,000) before we left Beijing. I can't stress enough that these are very honourable and very likeable people.

Cathy was her usual bubbly self, and we talked with her about seeing the Great Wall of China. She told us of a couple of places that are good to visit and said she could arrange a tour guide and driver for us. We chose a place to go and decided to go on Thursday, so we booked her guide.

We also wanted to go and see the Chinese Opera and we talked about the best way to do this too.

Then we asked about where we could get some Chinese food and she suggested she could order a takeaway for us. How about that, a Chinese takeaway in China!

We ordered Kung Po chicken and some ribs (They didn't know what prawn crackers are, so I am wondering if this is a British adaptation like Chicken Tikka Masala in Indian takeaways!) and egg fried rice.

The takeaway was delicious! It cost about £10 and was more than enough for the two of us. It also arrived about 20 minutes after we ordered it, so that was amazing too. I just hope it didn't come from the poisonous looking café around the corner!!! Still, even if it did, we survived and it was incredibly good to eat. Seriously, I think the takeaway did not come from the Bubonic Plague café, as Cathy was concerned to only send us to places she trusted and I don't think she would buy from there herself.

An eventful day came to an end with the now usual routine with the nurses. They were becoming friends with us and began to put in a bit more effort at English and teaching us some Chinese and having a bit of a laugh and joke with us – within limits and very respectfully.

Thursday 29 November

Thursday morning started as previous mornings.

Dr Dhu came in first and checked on me and confirmed that they needed to take the blood for the 2nd potential cycle of CIK.

The nurses arrived next, and did their observations and then set me up with my TCM drip. Meanwhile, Sheena made breakfast, scrambled egg with the beautiful bread we bought the previous day – Amazing!

Dr Zhao had been in every day (except the weekend) and sometimes twice a day with his entourage, making sure I was OK. He is very caring and we were also building a rapport with the other these doctors, Nelson Dhu has a good sense of humour and Yu Tao, a petite lady doctor, also very funny and personable. I was growing to like all of them.

I was feeling a little dizzy on this day and mentioned this to Dr Yu, along with a strange phenomenon which was that my elbows had gone black. No – it was not dirt! The skin had gone black on both elbows.

They were unconcerned about this and really did not do anything other than say it was not important. They were more concerned about the dizziness and took my blood pressure more often, but it passed and I was OK.

We went for a walk and as we were walking along by a car park, we noticed that several doors were open on a building that was in the car park. This turned out to be a public toilet with a number of cubicles that open straight off the road. It looked quite modern from the outside. Inside, it had toilets that reminded me of the latrines at school camp in some of the cubicles and some that were the same as the old French toilets that were essentially just a hole in the ground with a foot placement on each side of the hole. We decided that no matter how desperate we were, we would not be going in there!

Had Cheese and Broccoli Pasta for dinner – Sheena had brought all of the makings with us. Isn't she resourceful? It was very tasty.

Then we had a relaxing evening and watched some videos on our iPads. It is interesting that all American news channels are blocked, along with the BBC and Google. There are ways around this apparently, if you are desperate, but we didn't bother.

Friday 30 November

Usual morning routine happened before the troupe of Doctors came in led, as always, by Dr Zhao.

They said that they were intending to take the 2nd lot of blood as discussed. I said I was feeling dizzy again which they put down to the Prostap injection.

The nurses came in and set up the TCM drip Had TCM. Blood pressure 145/88

After the drip completed, they took everything down and the canula out.

We left the Hospital and walked a long way to the Hon Quai pearl market. It was not as exotic as it sounds and we were a bit disappointed with it. It all seemed a bit "Del Boy" inside.

There are also, McDonald's, Burger King and KFC here! What a bore.

Had a coffee in Starbucks though, before heading back to the Hospital. It tasted exactly how a Starbucks in London would taste, very good.

We bought some more lovely cakes and bread.

The school close to the Hospital and Temple of Heaven was turning out when we got there and we saw the children being met by parents and grandparents. Something else that is universal! There was also a street vendor selling glace cherries on a yew stick. Delicious!

Cathy came in and we had another nice chat with her. She suggested a takeaway of Chinese Dumplings and some Noodles etc. which we had but we were not so keen on this one. Still cheap enough at about £15 but we had some ribs with this too.

But an uneventful day drew to a close and we read and slept.

CHAPTER 15

Grand Opera - Chinese style

Saturday 1 December

Awoke at usual time with cleaners coming in but I felt really tired as I had not slept well. We decided to have a restful day in, reading. The temperature outside was dropping fast but the sky was still clear and bright.

I had taken John Steinbeck's "The Grapes of Wrath" which I found riveting and moving and was enjoying this today.

Sheena cooked breakfast of a ham omelette with bread. I have to say, the dried egg is really so good and made for some lovely breakfasts.

Cathy had arranged for us to go to the Chinese Opera that evening and a lovely lady met us in a car with a driver to escort us there. The lady's name is Yoyo. She was very charming and when we got to the theatre, she showed us all around and told us about points of interest.

There was a really nice souvenir shop there where we bought some gifts for friends and family including a couple of stunning paintings on ceramic tiles.

If, my Brother in Arms, you like Opera, beware - Chinese Opera is nothing like an Italian Opera, so clear that from your mind and prepare for something completely different. Proceedings opened when a man entered the stage and sat at a dressing table to demonstrate how the extremely elaborate makeup is applied.

There are several very clearly defined characters in every Chinese Opera and you can tell them apart by their makeup. This guy started by painting his face white. Then he applied some dramatic black markings and other painted details.

When this lengthy process was complete, he stood up and moved centre stage and some aides brought on a couple of mobile rails of dramatic garments and started to help him into them. There were many layers to this costume and it must be extremely hot under it all, but he looked very imposing and a little scary when it was done.

The Opera itself started and there is an electronic display showing supertitles and narration in English as the Opera proceeds. This is essential if you are to have any idea at all of what is going on! There is also an orchestra made up of traditional Chinese instruments and the music is exactly what you would have expected from the time of the Ming Dynasty.

The Opera is simple stories and when things happen it is as basic as "the soldier is walking along the road – he comes to a cross roads. He wonders which way to go" and he does elaborate "looking" gestures with his hand to his forehead as if shading his eyes which he repeats in each direction just so you get the point! Later there is a fight scene which takes place in the dark (there is a little light so the audience can see, but the implication is that it is pitch black) This is both extremely acrobatic and very funny (intentionally funny) if a little over-long as the joke wears thin after a while.

We were bemused by the story and the whole tenor (no pun intended) of the performance, but were glad we went. The leading lady sang a stunningly beautiful song – easily the most moving moment of the whole performance, and this went on while other ladies were wafting lengths of gossamer silk around the stage. It was a gorgeous sight and sound with the Chinese orchestral music.

Yoyo escorted us back to the Hospital and left us at the gate. A lovely evening and a lovely lady. If you like to experience other people's culture, then I would highly recommend it, but go with an open mind, and a willingness to let yourself go with it – I guarantee you will not have seen anything like it before. I was very tired and went straight to bed when we got back.

CHAPTER 16

The Great Wall of China

Sunday 2 December

I had requested that my TCM came early on Sunday as it was the big day – The Great Wall of China visit!

Following breakfast and the TCM we got ready and were met by our guide, Wallace, with a car and driver, all arranged by our wonderful coordinator, Cathy. Wallace had brought with him a number of bottles of water for us – very thoughtful of him and very welcome at times – the temperature had plummeted now and was below zero so we were well wrapped up.

We were driving for some considerable distance and left Beijing itself behind after travelling some rough and very rough roads that appeared as if we were heading into the country via farm tracks. We arrived at a factory with some coaches outside. Obviously, a tourist destination I thought. It turned out to be a Jade factory.

Inside were some amazing things and we received a demonstration of how they work Jade which is an extremely hard stone. Craftspeople working at machines were making the iconic balls within balls from solid blocks of Jade. We also learned about the different colours of Jade and were shown some truly amazing sculptures made from solid blocks of this beautiful material. Then, inevitably into the showroom where you can buy souvenirs.

Jade is expensive and the price is governed by the colour of the stone, as well as the size and complexity of the object. For example, a Happiness Ball is carved from a single block of Jade and consists of elaborate lacy design balls within balls. These are very expensive. We purchased a traditional green dragon in a medium complexity design. It was about £80 but is a nice souvenir for sure.

We had lunch at this place which was a buffet consisting of a huge variety of dishes from around the world – or at least, an approximation of dishes from around the world. Some of it was truly delicious, some less so. But nonetheless, we enjoyed it. I have to say we were not expecting lunch to be included.

Back in the car, we went a little further on back roads before finally emerging onto a very nice road that started gently snaking upwards until we were in the lower reaches of the clouds (It was a cloudy day, but we were also gaining altitude pretty fast in some places).

Finally, after about an hour and forty-five minutes we could see the wall on the hillside to our right. What a momentous sight. This is an international Icon and a treasure belonging to the world, not just to China.

The Great Wall of China was declared one of the New Seven Wonders of the World in 2007. UNESCO state that it is the largest man-made structure on Earth. The wall is made of a variety of materials, including packed earth, stone, brick and even wood. Much of the structure dates back to the Ming Dynasty.

The Ming dynasty sections of the Great Wall were built in the 1400's using a mortar composed of sticky rice flour and slaked lime. It is truly incredible that so much of the wall is still standing and is testament to their building skills and the durability of the materials and mortar selected. It is believed that more than a million workers died in constructing the wall although it is, apparently, not true that dead bodies of builders were built into the wall.

This is the largest man-made structure in the world and stretches (or rather snakes as it doubles back on itself in many places) for some 16000 miles.

The sight of this ancient wall was, for me, utterly breath-taking. I was stunned and entranced by it and felt that it was an absolutely magical place, full of history.

Wallace bought our tickets for us - they are very cheap by UK tourist attraction standards. Incidentally, many people claim that you can see it with the naked eye from space, but this is not true. You can't even see it from an airliner at 40,000 feet! Wallace showed us the way to access the wall, and then went back to wait for us in the car.

We climbed up some modern steps to get us to the height of the first tower and then looked out onto the wall itself which was snaking up the hillside ahead. We set off and soon made it to the first flights of steps of the wall itself. These steps are not built to modern building standards and range in height from a matter of 10cm to 35cm and in tread depth from 15cm to 50cm. Some of them are also severely worn so it is a fairly treacherous climb in places. It is remarkably taxing to climb such uneven steps. In some cases, you are climbing at an angle I would estimate at 70 degrees and I for one, felt the need to hang onto the steel handrail (which I suspect is a modern addition and not a relic of the Ming Dynasty).

The Wall vanished into cloud and mist and it was fantastically atmospheric, looking ahead at towers looming in the mist. Parts of the wall are semi-permanently closed, maybe for restoration work, I'm not sure. Anyway, it was an arduous climb to the farthest tower we could see and access, and it was very high.

Imagine my disappointment when we arrived and found that inside the tower was a souvenir shop selling the most tacky and cheap souvenirs. They looked like they were made in China! Oh – yes, silly me, they were! Nothing worth buying sadly.

This also marked the end of the section of wall we could access, but it was about an hour's climb to get there.

Heading back down was, in the steepest places, even harder than climbing up, but the views were amazing.

Looking at the wall itself, the blocks are stuck closely together and it is amazing to think that they used sticky rice in the mix and it is still there 600 years later and not even in disrepair. It is a worthy national monument to a great civilisation and I felt privileged to be there.

But this is not simply a tourist guide, there is a reason I am telling you all this about our sightseeing.

Yes, my Brother in Arms, you have to be pretty fit and well to do this climb which is remarkable for a stage 4 Metastatic Prostate Cancer sufferer in the course of treatment. I put it down to the TCM which makes you feel a million dollars, coupled with a determination that I was going to see this incredible wall.

Arriving back in the car park there were two parties of school children there of about 12-14 years of age and they surrounded us asking us to speak English with them, autograph their school pads and write things in English for them. They were so polite and charming. It was a delightful experience for us and they wanted photographs of us taken with them by their teachers. What a lovely experience with these open and friendly people. All of the children have at least some English – it is truly amazing!

Our guide provided bottles of water for us very considerately. We left there but I couldn't help staring at the wall until it was out of sight. We headed back into Beijing.

A little way into the city, we stopped again at a tourist spot. This time it was a Tea house. We were ushered upstairs and into a replica of a very ornate Chinese Tea House and invited to sit on some cushions, which we did.

A Chinese lady came in and started telling us about all the different teas and what made each one distinctive and more, or less, expensive than others. She made us little cups of tea in handleless cups. Some were amazingly good. Ginseng tea, Fruit tea (nothing like the concoctions you get in the UK called fruit tea – these had real fruit in them) Ginger tea, lychee tea, and a tea that is extremely expensive that comes in a small hard block like an Oxo cube.

After this, we were shown into an area where the teas and accoutrements were, inevitably, for sale. The prices, as in the Jade shop, are allegedly controlled by the government itself and we were advised that because of this they are fair prices.

Fair they may be, expensive they certainly are. Still, we bought a few small tins of tea and some bits and bobs. Very enjoyable.

Back in the car, we headed back deeper into Beijing before stopping again, this time at a silk factory! We were shown to a lift and taken upstairs where we received a demonstration of the silk craft from beginning to end. Seeing silkworms on Mulberry leaves (the only thing they eat) silkworm cocoons etc. and then being shown how the silkworm dies and it is the cocoon that is taken to harvest the silk. These are soaked in water and a thread teased out of them and hooked up to a machine, so as the water loosens the fibres it is wound onto the machine and the cocoon bobs around in the water held by this single continuous thread.

After this, they take you into another area and show how the raw silk is the worked to make it either into garments, or quilts or pillows. What is incredible is how much this amazing natural fibre will stretch – you simply can't break it. It will stretch and stretch and stretch. They let you have a go which is really interesting and fun.

Finally and inevitably, you are shown into the area where they sell silk goods and they talk you through the various qualities. There is literally something to suit every pocket in this place and again the prices are, allegedly, government controlled.

We bought a couple of silk pillows and some gifts for the family and considered some silk ties for the guys in the family, but held off thinking we would look elsewhere. I noticed the guide talking to one of the senior people at the silk factory and clearly talking about some sort of commission which I thought was fair enough.

Finally, our guide got us back to the hospital and I must admit I was pretty tired by then. We had paid £60 for the driver and guide for the day, which considering we had done probably about 160 miles or more and had the two of them for the day was amazing. He started talking to me about the possibility of a tip for the driver and suggested a figure that was about £10. I happily parted with £20 each for them thinking it was great value at a total of £100 for the two of them all day plus the car and its fuel – it was incredibly cheap. They were both very happy.

Back in the Hospital, we were both exhausted and had some more Pasta and retired to bed to read.

We both slept well.

CHAPTER 17

CIK Day approaches

Monday 3 December

The new week started in the same way as usual – Cleaner, Nurses for blood pressure etc. Then again, the Nurses with the TCM. Usual routine but by now I had discovered how to control the speed of the drip and I speeded it up so it only took just over an hour. The nurses looked a bit surprised that it was finished so soon when Sheena went to get them to take it down.

Dr Zhao and his team came in. Nothing much to report.

Omelette for breakfast – very nice. Sheena was egged out though and went for Granola (also brought from the UK).

We went for a long walk but in the general direction of the lovely cake shop where we bought more cakes and French bread. It was now bitterly cold – the temperature had plummeted to well below zero, but we had gone prepared for this and were enjoying the walks under bright clear blue, cloudless skies.

When we got back to the Hospital Dr Yu looked in on me. Had a lovely long conversation with her again ranging across many subjects including one of my favourite subjects – food, and specifically local Chinese food. She is a truly delightful and interesting person.

Cathy came in later and we opted for another takeaway, but given that we were not too keen on the dumplings, we reverted to the Kung Po Chicken.

<u>Tuesday 4 December</u>

Thirteen days into my adventure and all is going well.

Usual routines continued including my TCM drip. I was feeling very well indeed and had lots of energy.

Dr Zhao and Dr Yu Tao came in again. No Cathy, but Dr Yu translated.

Dr Zhao said that the CIK culture was growing very well and they would be ready to bring the treatment forward to Thursday. This was great news for me, I was really excited.

Dr Zhao also said it would be important for me to have scans done in the NHS after 3 months and to get them to him so he could check on the effectiveness of the CIK Immunotherapy.

They said my blood pressure was a little high at 145/88 but not too bad by my standards.

At this point, the little troupe of nurses came in to take the blood as agreed. The same routine was followed with the keen attention to sterilising the arm and everything surrounding it. The blood was taken, the same quantity as last time.

After this, we went out for a walk to the square again to watch the kites. The temperature was still falling and it was bitterly cold.

That evening, Sheena made Chicken with noodles and then settled down to watch a video and read.

<u>Wednesday 5 December</u>

The big day had arrived – CIK Immunotherapy day!

It started off much as all the other days with the routine of cleaning, nurses doing my temperature (and Poo Poo question) etc. as usual.

Then the nurses with my TCM came in and set up the IV for this.

The drip lasted an hour and a half as usual, give or take.

Then the senior nurse and another nurse came in and took down the spent TCM bag and hung a different bag on the hook with a clear liquid in it. I asked what it was.

She told me (in broken English) that it was an anti-allergenic drug in saline. This also lasted about an hour and a half.

Then Dr Dhu came in with the nurses and a trolley with the magic solution in it. The CIK!!!

They set this up in place of the anti-allergenic which was now finished.

I was elated and felt that this should have some sort of ceremony to it, but no – they were very matter of fact.

Dr Dhu explained that they had cultured the number of cells to 3×10 to the ninth power. This is three billion cells. It was not much to look at – about 250mls of normal medical grade saline solution.

I asked him how they knew there were 3 billion cells and he said he had personally counted them and that's why I hadn't seen him for a couple of days! We had a laugh. He is a great guy.

Following this drip (which I was sad to see finish) they replaced the bag with another bag of saline solution.

Throughout this process, they were carefully monitoring my temperature and blood pressure, both of which were steady.

So, that was my day – all taken up with having this procedure but I was absolutely thrilled that it had now been done and I visualised my little fleet of hunter killer submarines seeking out and killing cancer cells. I was willing them on!

I was feeling very tired, but otherwise very well. Tired, I suppose, because it was exciting to finally get the treatment I had come for and for which so many people had made so very much effort for me.

I slept very well that night.

Thursday 6 December

Woke up to the usual routine. Nurses paid careful attention to my temperature but it was 36.5 so normal.

Blood pressure good at 138/74 - Everyone happy.

I had my TCM drip and breakfast.

Nice chat with Cathy. Earlier in the week she had recommended HotPot.

The thing we found was, that the more we did that they had recommended, and the more we enjoyed it – the more enthusiastic they became in recommending things for us to try. This was a great thing to learn – note it well my Brother in Arms.

Apparently, HotPot is a big thing in China and a major social event for families. Dr Yu Tao had also mentioned this as something we should do.

I was imagining something from Coronation Street – like Betty's Hotpot, but this is not – repeat not, *anything* like a British Hotpot. You could not get further from that!

Cathy explained that the best HotPot restaurant is inside a shopping Mall in central Beijing. She said she would arrange a taxi for us when we wanted to go. We decided to go that evening.

I was absolutely fizzing with energy today – Sheena said I was bouncing off the walls, I literally could not sit still and I felt fantastic.

We had ordered a large cake for the staff from the western bakery which we had ordered with "Thank you" in Chinese and English on it. It was a big gateau and we hoped they would like it.

When we got back, we took the cake to the Nurses station and they were all excited. They wanted to take lots of pictures of us with them and we took some too. It was a lovely moment.

In the early evening, we asked Cathy to get our taxi, which she did.

We drove through the streets of Beijing again and it struck me it would be the last time, and I was wanting to take it all in. The taxi dropped us outside the shopping mall and we went in.

This place was huge – really huge! There were all kinds of shops in here, but they were all classy. Modern young people's clothes, electronics, watches, phones, jewellery, Ladies outfitters, Gentlemen's outfitters. Lingerie and all the big designer brands, Gucci, Fendi, Lacoste, Boss etc. etc.

We made our way up to the top floor where the HotPot restaurant is. This was another experience!

We asked for a table and were asked to wait outside where there is a line of chairs for people to use whilst waiting for a table. As we were sitting there for maybe 15-20 minutes, they brought little snacks and drinks for us, little packets of crispy things and soft drinks. It was all very nice.

Then we were asked to go inside and were shown to some soft seating, but still not into the restaurant. But here a man came along in a costume similar to the Chinese Opera and entertained everyone. He was great and gave us some little souvenirs, dangly things with painted faces one them like the Chinese Opera. Nobody else got these, so I suppose he spotted we were tourists (not hard, we were the only westerners there!). Then we were taken into the restaurant and shown to a table. This was a large square marble table with a big square hole in the middle and a hot plate set down inside the cut-out.

I had not the foggiest idea what to do. However, a waitress came over and introduced a young guy who spoke some English and he said he would help us. He explained that you order "Soup" to go in the middle of the table and you can have one, two or four different soups, spicy or mild.

We opted for one spicy and one mild mushroom – a good decision as it turned out as the spicy is *very* hot. Very nice, but very hot – I mean so hot your lips feel fat!

Then he explained that you order plates or half plates of various things, such as prawns, lamb, pork, beef or various vegetables such as spinach and bean sprouts and, of course, noodles.

We made some selections that he approved of and waited. The soups came very quickly and were soon followed by the plates we had ordered. The meat is raw and cut very thinly, and the idea is (as he showed us) that you drop them into the soup and they cook – pretty fast as it turns out.

You then scoop some out and into your dish, along with some noodles and some dips and salad stuff that you get from a buffet bar. Some of the dips are also very hot, but some are amazing – like the peanut one for example – I loved it.

You then eat this lot with chopsticks. There is no option on a fork or a spoon, so just get stuck in.

To drink, alcohol is not really the thing, but they suggested plum juice which was absolutely delicious!

It was all great fun, we loved it in here and the staff found it amusing but seemed to enjoy serving us.

This was another inexpensive experience, costing only about 175 Yuan again - £20. Yet another success to Cathy with help from Dr Yu!

When we finished, we went to another floor in the mall that had lots of baby and children's stuff and bought some things for our impending grandchild. They had lovely stuff here, much of it made in countries like Denmark and France. It was fairly pricey but very, very nice stuff.

After this, we left the shopping mall to go back to the Hospital.

This was a major challenge. Taxis do not seem to stop if you try to hail them and it took us more than half an hour to finally get one, by which time we were frozen. The temperature was displayed on the mall – minus 10 degrees and there was a howling wind as well!!

Glad to be back in the Hospital, we soon snuggled in for the night.

CHAPTER 18

Winding down

<u>Friday 7 December</u>

Woke up at around 06:45.
The usual routine continued, cleaner, nurses in to say good morning, nurses in to set up TCM drip, breakfast cold shower etc.

The nurses came back in and wanted more photos together with us which was lovely. Included Dr Zhao, and Dr Yu Tao in these pictures but Dr Dhu wasn't in today.

Dr Zhao (Professor Zhao) led my last consultation. Cathy and Dr Yu translated, but essentially, he was of the strong opinion that I should continue with both Bicalutamide and Prostap for the time being.

He reiterated that I should have scans in three months and that he would like to see them. For me, it was taken as read that I wanted him to see them.

Felt really tired today, but Cathy stayed on for a lengthy chat. We knew she did not normally work on weekends, so we gave her a bottle of designer perfume that we had brought from England (we thought we might need a few gifts so we had gone prepared) in case we didn't see her again. She was delighted.

Cathy and Dr Yu had both recommended that we see the Hutongs – a major tourist area, so we asked Cathy to organise a Taxi for us for Saturday.

We did go out, even though I was tired. We had seen a museum of natural history and thought it would be a good place to visit. It turned out to be mostly for kids, but there were some good dinosaur animatronics there and some really good dinosaur skeletons of animals I had not seen before.

Temperature was a tad warmer at minus 7 degrees, but still it felt very cold.

Saturday 8 December

Awoke at 06:30.

Usual routine including the Poo Poo question at which the nurse laughed – she was teasing me!

The nurses came in with my last TCM drip as we were leaving early next morning. I felt good today and was ready for our trip to the Hutongs – whatever this might be!

Over breakfast, Sheena read our guidebook about it to me. It is an area where the housing was of high quality and was designed for government and military officials of high rank. It is set around a large lake which I think is man-made, and has an area of shops and restaurants and also street food.

We signed out and left to get into the Taxi.

It was a shortish ride and we arrived at one end of the lake. It was very frosty and cold at minus 10 degrees again, but it made the lake and the trees very beautiful.

We walked for some way around the lake, stopping to take pictures and look at the houses.

A Rickshaw pulled up beside us. Now when I say a Rickshaw, it is not the kind with two poles and a little man with a Coolie hat running along pulling you to your destination. It is a more modern take on this, with a man on a bike which is part of the Rickshaw and instead of running, he pedals you along.

He offered us a tour of The Hutongs and, as he spoke good English, we accepted. It was very nice inside the Rickshaw with a lovely padded seat and it was all lacquered and decorated in Chinese style (what else?). We got in and he tucked us in with a blanket which was very welcome as it was very cold. He then offered to take our pictures using our phones.

This was a very informative trip and we are glad we took it. He showed us all around the back streets (which are very nice – not at all run down) and told us how you can tell how high ranking the official that lived in the houses would be. This is by the number of decorated beams that project over the front door. The more beams, the more important the resident.

He also took us to a house that was open to visitors. It is still decorated and furnished as it would have been when it was built, and you realise how relatively sophisticated these people were at the time.

He then took us to another place which we also went into and saw some other interesting things. There is so much to do that it was a pity it was so cold; I would have liked to walk around this place.

Our tour came to an end after about two hours, but it was well worth doing and not terribly expensive but definitely more tourist prices than local prices. Our guide was great.

He dropped us at a modern café where we had delicious hot chocolate.

After this, we were heartened for further sightseeing. We found a large building with various shops and restaurants inside as well as some street vendors selling hot food. I bought some barbecued chicken on a Yew stick skewer. It was absolutely delicious! Sheena bought a bag of miniature crabs fried in batter in a paper cone – like a bag of chips might be in the UK. They too were very tasty albeit a little crunchy.

This place was very beautiful and very different to anything else we had seen and, once again, we were grateful to Cathy and Dr Yu for recommending it.

We were both pretty tired so we decided to head back, especially as it was getting colder and also getting late in the afternoon. I found a Taxi and negotiated that he should use the meter – again he was not particularly happy to do that. If you go, my Brother in Arms, beware of this – a taxi can cost you a lot of money if you don't insist. One driver wanted to charge us the equivalent of £35.00 for a journey that had cost us £3.00 the week before!

Back at the hospital, we had some food and then set about packing as we had to leave the following morning quite early for our flight.

CHAPTER 19

Homeward bound

Sunday 9 December

Awoke at 06:30 and had final breakfast quickly, then showered (a hot shower as we were early into it! Actually Sheena always had a hot shower as she was always early, but I was always held up by the TCM!)

We did our final bits of packing and that was that.

Cathy came to our room to meet us and had a man with her to take our cases.

Gave gifts to one or two of the nurses we had had more to do with and a monetary tip to our cleaner who seemed very pleased. It was not that much to us 200 Yuan, about £25.00, but was probably a lot to her.

We also left some M&S chocolates and sweets and shortbreads from England (in England themed tins) on the Nurses station for all to enjoy. They were very happy with these too.

We went out to leave but the Nurses wanted more pictures by their station. They seemed like old friends we had been visiting!

We got into the car and started the 45-minute trip back to the airport and Cathy was very chatty with us telling us many things about herself and her family. The former policy in China (now abandoned) of allowing only one child per couple had led to many big problems as there are now many more men than girls so there is a huge imbalance in the population. The policy is now revoked. Social engineering is fraught with difficulties!

Chinese girls are now under pressure from their families to get married and have babies as soon as possible.

When we arrived at the airport, Cathy saw us right to the gate where she gave us big hugs and waved us off.

The flight home was on a Boeing 777 – nice but not as nice as the Dreamliner and it was a much busier flight, so we couldn't stretch out. Hey Ho.

I was amazed again at the vastness of both China and Russia as I followed our progress on the map. We also had the curious experience of chasing the sun around the globe as we crossed time zones and it never got dark outside.

Whilst on the flight, I reflected on my experiences in China which, I have to say, is a truly uplifting and inspiring place to visit.

Sheena and I had several very endearing encounters with groups of school children who would rush up and start saying the English words they had learned at school. They would also ask us to sign their little notebooks or anything they had – we were like rock stars! What they were doing was getting us to write English characters because it is, obviously, as foreign to them as Chinese characters are to us and to see somebody write it is fascinating for them. Several times, we were stopped for group pictures with them which were taken by their teachers, but this was a beautiful experience – they were utterly enchanting, absolutely polite and just so excited to meet us. Actually, I found the ordinary Chinese people to be very charming and extremely friendly. There is no guile to the ordinary people, what you see is what you get. I loved them.

We enjoyed good service from BA again. Finally, we left Russian airspace, into Scandinavia, across the top of The Netherlands and Germany over the North Sea and down into Heathrow to land at 3pm.

My brother-in-law, Ian, was there to meet us and we sped home to Hillingdon. It was lovely to see everyone but we were very tired and soon they left and we went to bed pretty early.

And that was that. The first leg of my exciting Cancer Journey was over. I hope you can see why I felt it was exciting.

But of course, it was not all over.

CHAPTER 20

Why can you not get this in the NHS?

Life returned to some sort of routine. I was now working, in the position referred to earlier, in Piccadilly as a Senior Clerk and travelling in on the tube every day, boarding at the second to last stop on the Piccadilly Line (Hillingdon) and going straight in to Green Park. It was an hour door to door. This is where my boss and the Barrister were raided by the National Crime Agency, you may recall!

All was OK health-wise, except that about two weeks after returning from China, I started to feel extreme fatigue in the afternoons. This lasted for about two weeks and then passed and I felt very well.

So, life went on as normal until March, when I had CT and MRI scans done by the NHS.

My next appointment with my Oncologist was a revelation.

She said "I have looked at your scans and I can see no tumour in the Prostate Gland, and the lymph nodes have shrunk to near normal size. I also cannot see any Cancer in the bones. She was definitely a little shocked at this result.

She talked for a bit more and then I asked her how good this result was on a scale of 1-10. Without hesitation she said "10 – definitely 10".

Frustratingly, she is still not interested in the CIK that caused this result!

I have however, since then, seen two programmes on TV, one saying they are using CIK immunotherapy, but only in conjunction with chemo and that they are using CAR-T Therapy but only on Leukaemia patients. Frustratingly, they followed three Leukaemia patients through treatment with CAR-T. But it soon turned out that instead of collaboration with the people who are already using it – they were starting from scratch – on the premise that British must be best, I assume. These foreign Johnnies cannot possibly have anything better than we have in the NHS!

All three patients died!

So although the NHS now proudly says it is using CIK and CAR-T Therapies, they say they cost the NHS some £200,000 per patient! This is an enormous sum of money and, frankly, if it genuinely is costing the NHS (and therefore you and me) this ludicrous amount of money per patient, then they/we are being royally ripped off!!

To carry out CIK immunotherapy of the kind they used on me in China, takes only a small and minimally equipped laboratory and a couple of Lab Technicians who are trained to separate the white cells, manipulate them to attack the Cancer cells and then create and feed the CIK culture.

This is not a drug, and therein lies the problem in my view. Big Pharma is not making money out of CIK and CAR-T and so they will almost certainly do everything they can to stop it happening in their biggest customers such as the NHS, especially as it offers actual cures for Cancers – unless of course they can get some business from it.

So, when discussing your treatment, never, for one second, lose sight of this paradigm. Big Pharma is a conglomeration of profit-making companies. They have shareholders who must be paid, so they are not there for altruistic reasons. They are not there to be your friend; they are there to make money. It may seem harsh to say but helping you is only a by-product of what they do and it is even arguable that their interests actually lie in NOT curing you.

Take for example, a patient on a standard Chemo therapy. What does this cost?

It is hard to isolate these figures, but I researched it online and estimates vary between £10,000 and £30,000 per patient per cycle of treatment depending on where you look. This is usually an 18-week cycle, so 18 doses of chemo will cost the NHS in this range – for one patient. How many cycles does a patient require? That depends, but it is usually several and sometimes many over the years.

The NHS spends £1.4bn that is £1,400,000.00 per year on chemotherapy alone. Where does that money go? Big Pharma. If they used CIK, how much of that eyewatering sum paid annually to Big Pharma could they potentially save? Certainly at least half of it and maybe much more – and Big Pharma would get none of it. Now you see why, I believe, Big Pharma would go to any lengths to stop it.

And remember dear Brother in Arms, I have just talked about the NHS here. What about all the other health services around the world that buy these poisons?

CIK by contrast, should cost next to nothing if each cancer hospital set up a lab and put in a couple of lab technicians. Big pharma would HATE this and trust me, they would put all kinds of obstacles in the way of the NHS doing this. Why? Because they would make no money whatsoever out of it, and it would prevent them from being able to continue selling expensive and poisonous chemotherapy.

Have you ever asked yourself this question?

When a business first brings out a new product – say for example, – a computer using some kind of new technology, they are very, very expensive indeed are they not? So expensive that most people cannot afford it.

But once rival companies start producing their own versions and the sales numbers increase, the prices drop and drop dramatically. Soon almost anyone can afford one and the companies have to look to their next product if they want to make the big money again.

Why does Big Pharma escape this rule of market forces?

Why is it that despite the fact that Big Pharma is producing millions upon millions of doses of these poisons every year and flogging them to the NHS (and others around the globe) – the price never, as far as I can tell, goes down. In fact, it goes up. The lame reason they offer for this is that it costs many millions to create and test these products and they have to make the money back somehow.

But think, my Brother in Arms, does this argument not apply in exactly the same way to say, computer technology? Sure it does, no question about it. Do the computer companies make money? Isn't Apple one of the richest companies on the planet? Yes – they make money alright - despite market forces that should apply equally to Big Pharma.

So why has Big Pharma been so successful in avoiding market forces and getting "clever" people including governments to believe that their business is an exception to market forces?

The answer, in the case of Britain, lies in the ridiculous fascination and trust the British people have in our sacred NHS. Politicians are scared to do anything that would cause an outcry regarding the NHS for fear of losing votes and you can be absolutely certain that if Big Pharma were threatened with market forces by a British government – they would make the mother and father of an outcry and, horror of horrors, politicians would lose their seats in parliament and Her Majesty's Opposition would capitalise on it like there is no tomorrow, under the banner of protecting the NHS and saving lives!

If I sound passionate about this, I am, and I make no apology for it. I attended a funeral last year (2019) of a good family friend, a truly lovely, lovely lady. She died of Bowel Cancer. Actually, that is not true – she died of Chemotherapy. The doctors admitted to her husband just before she died that the Chemotherapy had finally destroyed her vital organs. And so, after a 12-year struggle, she succumbed - to chemotherapy!!

Think about it - my friend that died of Chemo, she probably had 6-8 cycles of Chemo in her 12 years of suffering, maybe more. That's at least £250,000 on one patient for Chemo alone, plus all the steroids to minimise the effect of the poisons, the doctors the nurses and the hospital time, the scans, the biopsies etc. etc. etc.

Think about this: Chemotherapy is poison – *that is the point of it*. Yes, it kills cancer cells, but it kills healthy cells too. That is why people's hair drops outs, their nails deteriorate and they feel sick etc.

The theory behind it is that it may kill the cancer cells before it kills so many healthy cells that the patient's vital organs are overwhelmed and they die. Sadly, as in the case of my friend, this is not always the case.

In what other walk of life would this be acceptable? What if the aviation industry said – well, when we service the engines on your holiday jet, we have to put some sand in them to clean them. Yes, we know it will kill the engine eventually, but we hope it will complete many trips before it is finished and we hope it will not kill everyone onboard!

Maybe, in the beginning, along with conventional radiotherapy (which follows a similarly flawed plan), it was the only treatment available and we were grateful, because there was nothing else, but now it is not and we should *demand* better.

Is it not interesting that it is only now, after many decades of Big Pharma flogging these poisons for cancer patients, that when treatments such as CIK and CAR-T and HiFu and Nano-Knife and Cryosurgery are becoming gradually more widely known hey presto - Big Pharma is responding?

And just how is Big Pharma responding? By making what they are calling "Targeted Chemotherapies". (I don't think you can get these in the NHS as yet, but trust me, it will come eventually so as to keep the NHS on board). Targeted Chemotherapy is where they check the DNA of the cancer cells in the patient and remove parts of the scattergun makeup of the chemical concoction so that it does not destroy certain healthy cells. So they can now make Chemo that does not make your hair fall out or destroy your nails or make you feel sick or some others out of a kaleidoscope of symptoms – if you can pay!

Does it cure cancer? Sadly, it is no better or worse at that than it was previously. Yes, it will kill cancer cells, of course it will, but it also kills healthy cells – maybe in smaller quantities than previously but it still does it. How many people on chemotherapy do you know that have been actually cured of cancer? Not that many.

One study I read shows extended survival rates are linked to the patient not having a gene called ERCC1 which plays a part in repairing DNA – including the DNA of the Cancer itself![7] Those who do not have this gene survived on average a little longer than those who do. But even so, the figures are depressing as this is post-surgery chemo and the 5-year survival rate improved in those without ERCC1 from 39% to only 47%.

At best, and even if your own body's natural DNA repair system is not working against the chemo, your chance of still being alive after 5 years is still less than 50/50. Are you willing to take those odds?

Does targeted chemo cost less as there is less chemical in it? No, it costs more as they make it more suited to each particular patient! Amazing eh? Sell less for more! Nice work if you can get it.

Am I passionate? – you bet I am – this is an outrage and must be exposed and stopped.

As for the claim that CIK costs the NHS £200,000 per patient - I have absolutely *no idea* how this could possibly be true. The truth is that they could send the patients to China even including paying their air fares and, based on my experience, they would save some £165,000 per patient per cycle of CIK. And, many, if not most of the patients would be **cured**.

What lunatic could possibly think this is not a good idea?

Could it possibly be Big Pharma who really don't want you cured for £35k, they want you dependent on their monstrously expensive drugs for the rest of your life?

Will organisations like the NHS ever sort this out? Not a chance all the time Doctors are held in the thrall of Big Pharma and "standard practice" – and if you still aren't sure of this, refer back to the case of Ashya King who was very nearly a victim of this despite a better treatment being available. Yes, they take the Hippocratic Oath that they argue prevents them from using untried methods, so what can be done?

---

[7] Article Information – Oncotarget 2017 Aug 15 8(33)55246-55264
Authors: Lanlan Yang; Ann-Marie Ritchie and David W. Melton – Edinburgh Cancer Research Centre

The solution of course is easy - send doctors and scientists to China to study it and see the results for themselves – and stop feeding our money to Big Pharma and making our patients suffer in the process – WAKE UP AND SMELL THE COFFEE!!! Here endeth my NHS rant – for the time being.

I have to fess up to something here. CIK Immunotherapy is still in its infancy. However, it is working and it is virtually side-effect free and it is curing people of many types of cancer. They are still learning about this and are improving techniques all the time as you would expect and, even at the Puhua Hospital in Beijing, I believe they are now using another therapy alongside CIK to increase its effectiveness. But …… if you are simply improving a technique that is already curing cancers – side effect free – WOW!

I am going to tell you an amazing experience. It occurred in March 2019, so keep in mind that it was <u>after</u> I had returned from China and so after I had had my CIK treatment in December 2019.

I met a man, quite by chance. I did not know him, had never met him before, knew nothing about him in fact I had never even heard of him. He was in London with his family for a few days holiday.

I am naturally quite a gregarious person and said hello to him and he responded in a friendly way. We got talking and I asked him why they were in London. He told me that they were sightseeing. He also told me that he travels regularly to London on business.

I asked him what business he is in and he told me he is in pharmaceuticals, but he elaborated and said it is a very specialised branch of pharmaceuticals and that he was working with Cancer therapies.

Naturally, my interest was piqued so I asked what sort of therapies and he said it is called CIK immunotherapy!

Now you see why I had to swear that this is true – you couldn't make it up could you?

I told him that I had returned from China only in December after just having had CIK immunotherapy. He asked what Cancer I have so I told him, Stage 4 metastatic Ductal Adenocarcinoma in my spine, pelvis hip and lymph system.

He asked where I had had it done, so I told him the Beijing Puhua International Hospital and he knew of this particular hospital.

He said (and this stunned me) "You'll be cured".

I said "You sound very confident".

He said "I am 100% confident – *I know you will be cured*".

Well, I had read about the astounding successes with CIK but still, even at this stage, I hardly dared hope for a cure. Then he said something that stunned me further: "We have cures – and I mean cures, not treatments, for most cancers now".

I asked him why we don't know more about this and his answer you can believe or dismiss as melodrama as you wish. I fully believe it. He said:

"If I went public with the information I have, I would be dead within three days".

His belief is that Big Pharma will protect its own interests at all costs.

Let me put a question to you and see what you think. If Big Pharma started offering actual cures for the major diseases, what would happen? Well, obviously, you may say, their market would expand very fast. Correct – initially at least. However, once cures became commonplace and anyone could access them – what would happen to their market then? Their market would obviously shrink, and the more life-threatening diseases they cured the more their market would shrink. In the end, they would put themselves out of business.

So my question to you is – where do you think their interest really lies? In curing people, or simply treating them? Perhaps this may explain why Chemotherapy has hardly changed in substantive terms for decades.

One footnote to my lengthy rant on Big Pharma. I joined the Cancer Research UK (CRUK) chat forums and was sad to see so many desperate people looking for hope. I posted a brief account of my experience with CIK immunotherapy. Not promoting it, I didn't even say where I had it done or what it cost.

I started to get a number of enquiries from people asking these questions – where? How much? How does it work? Etc. I started to answer some of these questions but then my account was blocked. Finally, I was chucked off their site altogether. No discussion, no right of appeal. Why?

When I checked, guess what? CRUK has substantial links with Big Pharma to the extent that they proudly name their collaborations with Pharma companies on their website and admit that they receive money when drugs come onto the market that they have played a part in creating. On one level this seems both logical and fair. On the other hand, could it cause a conflict of interest when people like me talk about things that Big Pharma are not involved in? You decide.

They said I was promoting an unproven treatment. But if they are, as they claim, promoting research into cancer, why are they not open to investigating things like CIK? Why is it that scientists employed by CRUK seem only to work in collaboration with Big Pharma companies and, given this connection, is it logical that they could remain impartial or objective when alternative therapies that do not involve Big Pharma are presented?

I am not suggesting, as CRUK protest on their website, that Big Pharma has the cure for cancers and is hiding it (this would be criminally unethical), but I am saying that there would seem to be every incentive for them to oppose technologies that they are not involved in and which do not involve drugs that they might develop/manufacture, as it could be argued it works directly against their commercial interests. Dr Vernon Coleman argues this case very effectively showing how initial payments from drug companies with a "shared interest" with a charity, may start making small payments, leading to bigger payments and eventually partnerships with the charity, leading to a conflict of interest and in turn the charity becoming little more than a mouthpiece for the drug companies involved.[8]

Incidentally, the CEO of CRUK Michelle Mitchell enjoys a salary of some £244,000 per annum as reported online and you can check this quickly and easily on Google.

---

[8] Food for Thought – Dr Vernon Coleman MB,ChB,DSc, FRSA (ISBN: 9781898947974)

The argument always advanced in justification of such a salary is that you have to pay at levels comparable to industry to get the best. Interesting then, that Boris Johnson was paid £150,000 per annum in 2020. A question that I don't think will get an answer easily is, ' how much of the CRUK CEO's salary comes from Pharma companies either directly or indirectly?'

CHAPTER 21

What about other treatments?

Before I tell you of the second trip to Beijing, I promised you a discussion of some of the other forms of treatment I came across at various stages in my journey. So before I go onto my second trip to Beijing, this is what I know:

Firstly, HiFu – High Intensity Focussed Ultrasound. This is what it says on the tin, Essentially, they use Ultrasound to destroy the cancerous tissue with, apparently, little or no damage to healthy tissue.

When I was researching for myself, I never came across this form of treatment and, in any event, I would not have been a suitable candidate due to the metastasis I had already suffered.

HiFu clinics are now easy to come across online, certainly on a private basis.

Can you get it done on the NHS? This is a slightly more difficult question. At the time of writing this, it is not available commonly through the NHS but there are some cases where the NHS might refer a patient to a private clinic for this form of treatment.

Once again, the NHS is so far behind the curve it makes one want to tear one's hair out. They say there is not conclusive evidence of the long-term success rates and so they are exercising caution. Whereas, for me, Chemotherapy has advanced comparatively little over the decades and hardly has a stellar record. So it seems to make sense to me even to the point of being the obvious thing to do, is to use some of these other therapies to try them out. For example HiFu which, given even short to medium term improved prospects, coupled with the fact that you could always revert to other treatments if HiFu did not work long term – why would you not do it?

Would there be willing participants? You bet there would. My two beloved Uncles on my dad's side, Peter and Bing (Eric), both died of lung cancer after many years of smoking. I visited them both and during these visits they begged, with tears in their eyes, for some treatment – even experimental treatment, to just be able to live another couple of years.

Once again, Big Pharma continues to benefit by the indolence of the NHS – it is like wading waist high through molasses in winter to get anything changed for the better.

The reported side effects, are few and minor and discussions of them are easy to find online. So, if you are interested and think you may be a suitable candidate for HiFu (i.e. the cancer is contained within the Prostate or other localised area) then I suggest you get researching on this as the position is changing fast all around the world.

One other treatment I wish to comment on is Rigvir. This is a viral treatment, (Oncolytic ECHO-7 virus) where a live virus is introduced to the patient's body. The virus has been modified so that it infects and kills cancer cells.

I have a friend who has had this treatment for advanced breast cancer. She and her husband travelled to Latvia for it where she also had CIK immunotherapy.

The results have been dramatic and in the last conversation I had with her husband, it seems she is very hopeful that she is cured.

Whether it was the Rigvir or the CIK that has produced this result, or indeed, a combination of the two, it is hard for me to say.

My only concern with Rigvir is that if you introduce a live virus into your body, what happens to it over time? Does it simply fade away, or does it remain in your body perhaps to awaken and produce effects that are unwelcome. Could you pass this virus on to others, for example unborn children and, if so, for how long could you pass it on and what would be the effects of this virus entering the system of a person without cancer?

For these reasons, personally, I would have chosen not to go that route unless and until all other preferred options had failed or been unavailable. As a last resort, I would certainly have considered it, and, should my cancer return, I may well consider it.

Once again, it is not available on the NHS although in this case, I can understand their reticence in bringing it forward for the reasons mentioned above.

And what about the Grape Cure?

This is undoubtedly worth a second look if you are faced with any sort of cancer at any stage.

If you can't afford to go to China or Latvia or other places for any of the other treatments, and you can't see any way to raise the money, then get the books mentioned earlier: The grape Cure by Johanna Brandt and The Grape Cure by Basil Shackleton.

I think almost anyone can afford to buy grapes and remember, you do not have anything else to eat or drink for 28 days – grapes – preferably with seeds, and pure grape juice, not from concentrate.

The accounts in these books are more than thought provoking, they are convincing.

Be aware, that the books state that you will feel *extremely* ill after a few days on the Grape Cure, but this is supposedly the grapes working on the ills in your body. The authors seem confident that you will survive and will probably be cured of your cancer.

You can be sure that, should my cancer return, I shall do the grape Cure.

As a final note on other treatments, I am not an advocate of recklessly introducing new treatments willy-nilly in the hope that some might work and produce favourable results.

I am, however, a passionate advocate of learning from others, which the NHS seems curiously opposed to doing. I don't know if it is the idea that unless it is British it can't be any good or that they fear that 'anything from these foreign Johnnies can't be all it's cracked up to be'.

Whatever it is, their tardiness with treatments that are gaining positive track records around the world is unforgiveable in my view. Especially so, in the face of the known harmful consequences of the treatments they persist with that are very difficult to live with and destroy people's quality of life and, ultimately in the case of my friend mentioned earlier who battled for 12 years against bowel cancer, destroys their life itself.

What is your view?

CHAPTER 22

Back to the future

Back to my Exciting Cancer Journey then.

I obtained copies of my latest scans although it took some time although I am not criticising the NHS over this, it was just circumstances. Eventually, I was able to send them to Professor Zhao.

He concurred with my UK Oncologist that some Cancer was still visible in my Lymph system and pelvis. He recommended going back for the second cycle of CIK.

I made arrangements to do this.

This time Sheena could not come due to commitments.

My Brother-in-Law, Ian said he would come with me so he obtained a Visa and we purchased tickets to arrive in Beijing in September 2019.

Monday 23 September

To Heathrow for the flight to China. We had booked Premium Economy seats to give a bit more legroom. These were very comfortable and we got significantly upgraded entertainment and food. Very nice. I would certainly recommend this if you intend travelling to China – it's a long, long way. Besides, the cancer on my left hip had started off osteo- arthritis and I was finding it hard to be sat for long periods in confined spaces.

Tuesday 24 September

We arrived in Beijing, not quite a year from my first visit. We were met at the airport by Ada. She explained that Cathy was on holiday and we might not see her. This was a bit disappointing, but Ada is very nice and very helpful too, albeit a bit more down to Earth and less "wacky" if I can put it like that - I mean wacky in the nicest possible sense – Cathy is just so much fun.

I had told Ian that I was amazed at how few accidents happened on these roads, given how close the Chinese drive to each other. No sooner had these words left my mouth, than he saw an accident, and another about 50 yards later! In fact we saw three in total on the way to the Hospital. Maybe my first impression was not accurate.

I noticed in the streets immediately surrounding the Hospital, where the derelict apartment blocks, I mentioned previously stood, that people had moved back into many of them! Still no windows or doors and presumably no power or gas, but such is the poverty I guess they were desperate for something, anything, to live in. I imagined, the amount of money I was spending to get well would be an immense fortune to them.

On arrival at the Hospital, everything seemed very familiar to me and we were shown to the same room that Sheena and I had shared.

The nurses all commented that I had put on a lot of weight. This was not good. I was definitely overweight and now even more so than last year.

In the room, Ian got the sofa bed! Well, I had to have the Hospital bed – I was the patient! Anyway, there is no doubt that the sense of propriety of the nurses would have dictated that they would have ordered me into the Hospital bed!

Dr Zhao and another Doctor whose name I never got, came in with several nurses, two of whom I recognised from previously.

He enquired as to how things were going for me and then set the nurses on me.

Blood pressure, temperature and Poo Poo questions already! In addition to this, they took six vials of blood for tests. Blood pressure pretty high and they tut-tutted at this.

They also came in with the TCM and set me up with a canula in my hand and fixed me up on a very welcome drip – this stuff is magical!

So, the routines that were so familiar were back in place immediately.

Later that day, they came to take me for a CT scan, complete with contrast injection.

Then an MRI scan.

The same routine as my last trip was followed with regard to the queue outside the CT and MRI scan rooms. Essentially, I was at the front of the queue every time!

After all this was done, Ian and I went out for a walk along the river eastwards but I was tired and could not go very far.

Wednesday 25 September

Ian took the role of Sheena in making food for us and made a delicious meal of scrambled eggs with granola afterwards. Very nice.

The nurses trouped in and seemed very happy to see me again. They went through the routines but were shocked at my blood pressure which was very high and would not let me leave the Hospital. They told me I had to stay in bed.

The nurses set up my TCM drip and I was, again, happy with that.

Ian went out to the supermarket by taxi and had some fun there. He came back with some bread amongst other things.

I felt extremely tired and had some severe pain in my left hip. To be honest with you, My Brother in Arms, and from a desire to hide nothing from you, I was fearful that the cancer was back and was responsible for the way I was feeling, both the pain and the tiredness.

I was feeling a lot less able than last time because the cancer on my left hip had set off a chain of events leading to severe Osteo-

Arthritis. This made it painful to walk on occasions and I was also getting back pains which made it hard to walk or stand for long periods of time. I would also become tired more quickly.

Dr Zhao and his new team came in with Ada to translate). He had the results of the new scans from yesterday and my PSA score.

PSA was 0.037. An amazing result!

He then said that they had carefully examined the scans and could not find any cancer anywhere. Not in my spine – and he said, using his fist cupped in his hand as an illustration, that the cancer was gone and had left a hole (he withdrew his fist) and that the bone of the vertebra was regenerating and the hole was getting smaller and closing up. He explained that the back pain was caused by the damage from the Cancer, but the cancer had gone.

I could not believe this news but he assured me it is true and the other Doctor (a lady) confirmed this. He also said that the lesions on my pelvis and hips had gone and that my Lymph nodes had returned to normal size and that there was no sign of Cancer anywhere.

This news was clearly amazing.

He recommended that, as the CIK was already prepared, that I should go ahead with this as an insurance policy but that the news was extremely good. He was very happy.

I agreed that we should go ahead with the second cycle of CIK.

So, that was that. I asked where Dr Dhu and Dr Tao were and they both, it seems, had taken up posts at other hospitals although Dr Dhu had taken the opportunity for a sabbatical as well. I missed them; they were great fun.

I was however, elated at the cancer news.

Thursday 26 September

Awoke at around 06:30 and Ian got showered and dressed in time before the cleaner arrived.

Shortly after this, the Nurses trouped into say good morning and then shortly after that the blood pressure, temperature and Poo Poo routine. Blood pressure just a little better than yesterday.

Shortly after that, the Nurses came in with my TCM and set up the drip. I was drawing a lot of comfort from this as it made me feel really good.

Ian made breakfast – I had trained him to do the scrambled egg the way Sheena did although he was much stingier with the butter because of how much weight I had put on!

Following this consultation and the drip finishing, we got ready and went out for the rest of the day. I was elated.

Previously, I had thought to take Ian to Tiananmen Square and The Forbidden City, but we were told it was all closed off to visitors for preparation for the 70th Anniversary of The People's republic of China celebrations. This was a disappointment for Ian as it meant he was so close but so far and would not get to see it at all.

We went to the Summer palace instead which I had not seen, so it was new for both of us.

He said he had been disappointed with his first views of China as he had not envisaged it as this at all. I think he had been expecting a romanticised view of it with misty willow trees, rivers and bridges with ladies in their elegant silk Kimono style dresses with fans and decorated sticks in their hair!

It is nothing like this now, it is a modern and thriving economy with all the modern trappings and accoutrements on display although there is some serious and grinding poverty clearly on view as well.

However, The Summer Palace takes you some way towards this idyll that my brother- in- law had envisaged.

This place is truly spectacular! Again, Ming and Qing Dynasty Emperors used this Palace and grounds exclusively for themselves and their wives and entourages. The gardens are gorgeous and the whole place is set around a huge lake with an island.

There are long covered walkways with lovely views of the lake and gardens and it is clear that this place was designed for relaxation and recuperation from the excesses of being Emperor, although it is so obviously luxurious that no doubt some excesses occurred here too!

Various little pavilions and mini-palaces are dotted around. And you can go into all of them.

We went across to the island on a boat (which was quite pricey) and frankly, I think it was hardly worth doing. What was on the island was not very dissimilar to everything else we were seeing.

Ian said this was much more like the China he had been expecting and it was true that it did conjure up images of armies of Coolies carrying a fleet of Litters with the Emperor, his wives and high-ranking minions hither and thither around this place.

It is truly beautiful here and the air smells so clean, I think because there are so many trees here – many of them scented varieties.

Unfortunately, after about three hours I became very tired and could not continue walking around. Ian very graciously said that he had seen enough anyway and wanted to visit the souvenir shop. This was a big cut above other souvenir shops we had seen and we both bought some nice things.

Back in Dongcheng, we saw a KFC and decided to go in. KFC is marginal for me at the best of times but, my Brother in Arms, I must warn you, I found it utterly disgusting. It was greasier than any KFC I have ever had before and had an unpleasant overtone of Chinese takeaway flavours to it all. Most of the chicken was not coated and the chicken wings were yellowish white and looked un-cooked! It was truly vile. The taste still haunts me today and I cannot now go near a KFC!!

Friday 27 September

Usual events unfolded up to and including TCM drip.

Dr Zhao and team visited but not much to report by him or to him.

We had booked a visit to the Great wall today and our car with guide was awaiting when we went outside. I had decided that it might be best to go to another section of the wall as we had been told there was more to see there than at the part Sheena and I had gone to.

This turned out to be true, but whereas Sheena and I more or less had the wall to ourselves, this section was swamped with tourists. It was like visiting a facsimile of the Great Wall at Disneyland! It was still worth seeing, but not as atmospheric as the last time I saw it. It was also September, so perhaps the tourist season was still in full swing whereas later in the year when it is very cold, maybe there are not so many tourists - this could account for the difference I suppose.

We did the same round of Jade factory, Silk factory and Tea House. Ian enjoyed this and bought some Jade for my sister-in-law as well as some silk pillows and duvets.

Another successful day.

Had a takeaway that Ada organised for us. Kung Po Chicken as recommended to Ian by me. It was delicious - again! Ian was happy!

Saturday 28 September

Nurses arrived and usual routine followed.
CIK was scheduled for the next day.
Stayed near the hospital, but we went for a walk along to the bakery where the gorgeous French bread is sold.
Back at the Hospital, Ian cooked some dinner using a tin of spam- like meat he had bought and the scrumptious bread. It was OK. He is a very resourceful man.
We settled in to do some crossword puzzles and then read before what, for me at least, was very welcome sleep.

Sunday 29 September

Awoke early again before the cleaner arrived. It gets light quite early in September.
The nurses followed the cleaner on the good morning routine, followed by the blood pressure etc. nurses, followed by the TCM.
Ian made breakfast. He had got the hang of scrambled egg using dried egg very early on and this was great.

An hour and a half later, they returned to take the TCM drip down and set up a saline drip.

They took my blood pressure and temperature again.

They returned when the saline drip had finished and removed it. The senior nurse was with them this time.

They took my temperature and blood pressure again.

They connected the bag containing the CIK and set it off.

I lay there contentedly watching the fleet of hunter killer submarines entering my system and willing them on again.

Dr Zhao and the lady doctor and Ada came into see me. We had a very pleasant conversation during which I asked him what my prognosis would be now. His answer is burned into my brain:

"Forget about Cancer, and live your life. You will die of something else now".

I asked him if I should return to China for another cycle of CIK at some point in the future. He shrugged and said "What for? the job is done!"

I wanted to make sure I got every drop and watched the line empty into my arm before calling the nurse to take it off.

They returned and set up a saline drip again.

This done, my treatment was finished!

Hurrah and Hurrah!! Now, I thought, I need to see the results.

Then Ada came in and asked if we were transferring to an Hotel as tomorrow was our last day in the Hospital. This was a bit of a bombshell as I had given them the dates of our flights and had not previously had any idea on which day I would be getting the CIK. As we were only in China for 8 days, I assumed it would be right at the end.

I told Ada what my decision-making process had been and that I had given Crystal my flight details and assumed the CIK would be at the end of my stay and had not planned to go anywhere else.

Later, she came back with a document and this showed how much we would have to pay to stay in the Hospital. It was quite a bit given that we were not expecting it.

We started to look at the price and location of Hotels and after about an hour, we found one close to the airport and were in the process of making a reservation when Ada returned and said she had spoken to the manager who said we could stay in the Hospital at no extra charge and they would transfer us to the airport for our flights.

This was a bit of a relief, but one disappointment, tomorrow would be my last TCM drip!

We went for a walk, but they were not keen on us going far from the Hospital as I had just had the CIK and everywhere was being prepared for the celebrations on 1 October.

Monday 30 September

Tomorrow was also 1st October which was the 70th Anniversary of The People's Republic of China, so I mentioned to Ada that we thought we might go to Tiananmen Square to watch the parades and displays.

She looked horrified and said "No! You must not do this; you would get into a lot of trouble!". Whoops! I suppose I had become accustomed to thinking that this is a free country since, apart from the petty direction that you must carry your passport at all times (which we did, even though I had only been asked to show it once – going into the Dinosaur Museum of all places!) but now it came home to me that this is after all China, a communist state and, if you are unwise enough to step out of line, there could be trouble.

We opted for discretion being the better part of valour.

Instead, we went for some walks along the river and planned an evening trip for HotPot as I had told Ian how great this was. I knew it would be right up his alley!

Ada had organised for us to have a Taxi and off we went.

I was disappointed to see we did not have to wait outside, as I think Ian would have enjoyed seeing what they do, but hey-ho, we went straight in and were seated at a table near the salad bar.

A truly delightful waitress came over and started talking to us in broken English about what we wanted. I think she must have liked us as she suddenly seemed to switch into gear to organise everything for us to get maximum enjoyment!

First, she brought us a plate with some slices of water melon, and this was very nice.

Then she took our order and I led the discussion somewhat as I at least knew roughly what to expect. We had the Mushroom soup and a spicy one again. And I made sure to order the prawns, beef and lamb and some vegetables.

The waitress directed us to the salad bar and we went to get some bits and pieces and some dips.

When she returned, she had a tray with some other dips on it which she explained were "on the house". Then she made a gesture for us to watch something and a waiter came out of the kitchen and picked up what looked like a small towel from a tray.

He started spinning this around and it began to stretch, longer and longer and then he divided it in the middle to create a loop and began swinging it around like a lasso! It must have got to about ten feet in length when he began performing all sorts of tricks with it swinging it up and down and round and round – it was brilliant.

He actually broke a couple of these, but binned them and continued with a new one until he did one perfectly and it was then cut into lengths. Have you guessed what it was? Noodles!!!

This was just amazing to watch, and entertained not just us but many others at tables nearby. He was very skilled.

The waitress continued bringing us little bits and bobs of food to try – she was truly exceptional and made us feel like royalty.

When we finished our meal, I asked for the bill, but instead she brought us a huge platter of fruit and candied treats. We were absolutely stuffed and had had so much fun.

When the bill came it was 175 Yuan – about £20 – the same as when Sheena and I went there, but we had had so much more!

We got a taxi back to the Hospital and settled in for the evening doing crosswords and reading.

A petite young nurse came in to take my blood pressure and she showed me the reading which was really high. I exclaimed "Whaaaat?" when I saw the reading. She looked really shocked and upset as if I thought it was her fault! I quickly tried to make her feel better, but she said she would come back in half an hour to do it again and that I should rest.

I did rest, but when she came back it was not much lower. It seems strange that when they do blood pressure, they only do it once, whereas, my experience in the UK is that they do it at least twice and take the lower reading. Still, it was high and that was that.

They did seem to look in on me a lot during that night!

Tuesday 1 October

Next morning awoke early, then cleaner, nurses and usual routines.

Ian and I went for a walk and noticed there were many police around. Little convoys of police motorcyclists were going along the highways and smaller groups of them were on the smaller roads that we were on by the river. None of them took any notice of us.

We went to the bridge close to where the ancient gate to Beijing is situated and looked in the general direction of Tiananmen square but, frankly did not dare to wander too far, for fear of getting noticed.

We mooched about and watched little groups of old men playing cards and Mah-jong.

When the festivities kicked off, we were back at the Hospital and turned on the TV to watch it, frustrated that we were just 6 kilometres from where it was all happening but were not allowed anywhere nearby.

When they started the flying display, we went outside to see if we could see the planes. We saw no jets, only helicopters trailing red smoke. This was good, but we hoped to see the fireworks later.

We heard a few bangs, but decided TV was the best option.

Wednesday 2 October

Got up early and finished last minute packing. We said our goodbyes and Cathy took us to the car and on to the airport.

It was a good, uneventful, flight back home on a Boeing 777 although I had tried to get us upgraded and was irritated that the flight attendant told me they had no upgrade availability then came and took two people who had entered the plane after us and were sitting behind us for….. would you believe it - complimentary First-Class seats! He saw me and looked a little sheepish. Blackadder expletive comes to mind.

BACK IN THE UK

I did not intend for this book to become a travelogue, and I hope you did not feel it was that. My thinking was that I felt it important to put my excursions in China in and show how physically demanding they were to demonstrate how well I felt throughout my treatment. I hope you found these sections interesting and amusing.

I have to admit to feeling somewhat cut adrift when my Chinese treatment was finally all over.

Back in the UK, it was hard to have to settle back into the general malaise I feel exists in the NHS over Cancer treatment.

Here I was, having had a radical form of treatment and saved the NHS many thousands of pounds in the process and they had no interest whatsoever even in seeing what the results were.

Frankly, I find this shocking.

My first consultation after my Chinese sojourn with my UK Oncologist was interesting. She is not willing to do any new scans unless and until my PSA starts rising rapidly.

She said, "when it returns, we will do some scans to see what is going on".

I said "You seem very sure it will return".

She said, "Oh yes, it will return – it always does".

Well. I guess we shall see.

So far so good though, I have no pain and no other indication that it has returned.

CHAPTER 23

Epilogue

So, My Brother in Arms, what will you do?

Obviously, I can't answer that question for you, even though I know what I would do in your position.

My view is that even if my Cancer were to return, the experiences I have had and the time without symptoms or chemo induced illness have given me time to build more precious memories. I would not trade this for anything. Especially not for months of illness and anguish and helplessly watching my life slipping away.

I have seen China which I always wanted to do – and, I must tell you, Sheena says very firmly that she is now very glad she went there, she enjoyed the experience enormously even though she had always said she did not ever want to go to China.

Keep in mind this fact too, Sheena was on a trip to get cancer treatment for her husband who was under a death sentence, and still she enjoyed the trip so much!

I have met some beautiful people in China, the Doctors (especially Dr Zhao, Dr Dhu and Dr Yu) and the Nurses and Cathy and Ada all have been truly lovely, as well as many others we just met in passing. I have seen some wonderful places and had wonderful experiences in China.

I have seen how much I am loved by my family and that gives one great pause for thought, I can assure you. In fact this is probably the greatest insight I have gained from this disease. I have enjoyed some very happy times with my family, and feeling well in those times which is beyond priceless when you have had a reprieve from a death sentence.

I have seen my precious little grandson, Vincent, born and am happily watching his progress through learning to walk and talk and calling me "Gan Gan" all whilst feeling well – so I can enjoy him to the full - what a delight!

The shocking reality is that if I had accepted the first offer of treatment with the NHS – Chemo – I would have been ill for possibly 6 months and by now simply awaiting, or more likely enduring, the return of the symptoms. I would now be two and a half years into a 3-year prognosis. I think 6 months would now be looking a very, very short time indeed from here! It would be like being one step from the top of the Gallows and just a couple of short paces from the noose.

Yes, I have, along with everyone else, endured the COVID-19 lockdown from March 2020 and, as I write, am enduring lockdown 2 in November 2020. This is not great as there is so much I still want to do, that the restrictions are almost unbearable.

But to think that this might have been my last few months of life trickling down the toilet if I had followed the NHS recommendation is shocking – just shocking!

Whatever choice you make, my Brother in Arms, and I mean this absolutely sincerely, make sure it is a decision both you, and your family can live with.

For me, deciding to go to China for CIK immunotherapy was one of the best decisions I have made in my life. It literally took me from a death sentence to The Great Wall Of China!

I am still on the Patch Trial at the Hospital in West London and still have my PSA score monitored. I am pleased to report there are no alarm bells ringing at this time!

I am still on Prostap injections, and Dr Zhao advised that I should stay on these permanently.

Do they have side effects? Yes, they certainly do. I am not sure whose bright idea it was to fill men up with female hormones but I assure you it has consequences.

Hot flushes for one, (I have developed huge sympathy for women in the menopause!) and I have become very emotional, I cry often and sometimes at little or nothing. There is also a risk of Osteoporosis and muscle loss, and you can grow tits - of which they tell you they can stop the development with radiation. BRILLIANT!! (doesn't radiation cause cancer?). As I said to my Oncologist and specialist Oncology nurse "I like breasts, I am truly a big fan of them, but I don't want a pair myself!" Oh and putting on weight is another consequence that is hard to deal with.

Your testosterone drops to extremely low levels – with further consequences I choose not to spell out to avoid my own pain. Use your imagination.

I hope for a better treatment than hormones to come along at some point but, if this is the price I have to pay for living longer to be with my amazing family and feeling well along the way, then so be it. But there is no doubt it impacts on your feelings of masculinity.

I was never a real he-man type but I enjoy being a man and everything that goes with being a man, except this I suppose – this, after all, is exclusively a man's disease.

So, in conclusion, the big question:

Am I cured?

Truthfully, I don't know. Dr Zhao thinks so and my Pharmaceuticals friend I met in London thinks so. But I no longer go along wondering about it, I simply get on with life according to Dr Zhao's advice.

Would I do it again from the same position I found myself in in June 2018?

In a heartbeat!

ENDNOTE - CREDITS

I would like to credit the many people who donated via GoFundMe and these are named below. And to thank you for the love and in many cases, the loving comments which continue to mean so much. And there were many more who donated directly to my bank and these too are very dear to me.

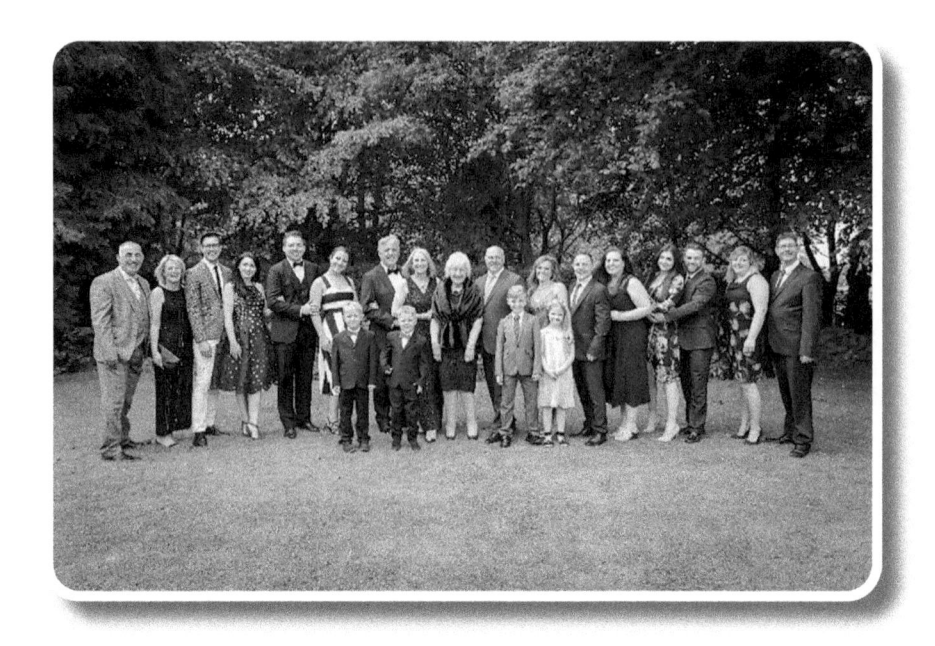

My Astounding Family pictured here (from Left to right)

Eddie and Caroline Kretay (Emma's parents)
Alex and Emma Hopkins
Aymeric and Eliza Robert
Me and Sheena
Madge Jackaman (my esteemed mother-in-law AKA Dame Edna)
Ian and Alison Jackaman (my brother and sister-in-law)
Adam and Lisa Jackaman
Chloe and Luke Jackaman
Becky and Kev Clarke

Front:
Alfie and Toby Clarke
George and Aaliyah Jackaman
(And not pictured here) – my dear little grandson Vincent Edward Hopkins

MY EXCITING CANCER JOURNEY

And my special thanks to:

Nigel and Chrissie Foster
Nathan and Rose Beehl
Clive and Sue Thomas
Guy & Toni Tarditi (& James Patrick Page)
Sebastien and Estelle Denny
Alain & Valerie Robert
Serge Robert
Antoinette Robert
Gary & Sammy Saunders
Sarah Thomas
Ben Thomas
Terry & Jo Worts
David Rose
David Goodman
Jess Sohal
Mike and Jean Taylor
Hayley Marsh
James Redjeb
Chloe Edwards
Richard Blackshire
Sophie Hermange
Daniel Amedoda
Carla Toro
Rosie Walker
James & Claire Burnett
Rebecca Unwin
Jersino Jean-Mary
Linferd Campbell
Andre Richards
She'miah Hastick
Fern Rhode
Sobia Kazmi
Alex Welsh
Edith Brockbank

Anon (JL)
Maija Hayward
Mitchell Smith
Debbie Temple
Eric Eamon
Jadine Eamon
Simon Temple
Ahsan Zaidi
Andrew Rasiah
Mihail Alberti
Susan Bartlett
Zuzana Gondova
Racheal Hicks
Michael Power
Kyle Barnard
Michelle Dye
Hannah Sweeting
Jane Swan
Jenny Giss
Lauren Kempster
Joe and Sylvia Rankin
Christine Cooper
Heather Watkins
Elizabeth Jacques
Graham Leslie
Sue Rothery
Mike Burke
Gavin Howes
Penny Rhode
Amy Simpson
Ian Williams
Ellen Nduka
Margaret Adams
Bethan and Abbie Moore
Asif Ansari (who inspired me to write this book)
Nye Nduka and family

MY EXCITING CANCER JOURNEY

Aaron George
Monica West
Richard Smith
Jo Barnard
Giuliano Antonucci
Luke Wainwright
Becky Money
Jade Jones
Alex Barnard
Chris Ash
Tom Paga
James Bennett
Victoria Hair
Laurence and John Denton
Nathan O'Looney
David Barnard
Nadine Stevens
Amina Syed
Richard Zunik
Garry Wilson
Joanne Couch
Elizabeth Gover
Victoria Yogendra
Marcello Cuconato
Thomas Kenward
Martin Kowalski
Mary Nahkala
Patricia Hurley
Sandra Hyman
Steve Mougoue
Buzz Seager
Sarah Buchta
Louis Brudenall-Jones
Gerard Doyle
Adam Pape
Adrian Wing

MARTYN HOPKINS

Ben Putman
LLorelei Henry
Friend of a Friend
Virji Owandji-Okutu
Claire O'Donohue
Chris Rose
Elle Taylor
Chloe Greener
Sophie Reid
Kira and Tom Clarke
Naomi Rothwell-Smith
Marina Chirco
Oliver Graystone
Warren Baldwin
Nicolas Bayle
Theresa Meck
Helena Roome
Richard Hughes
Sue Thomas
Toby Sampson
Lynda Walker
David Oddy
Louise Welsh
Patrick Ntienou
Despo Bains
Salima Ali
Heather Breith
Jennifer Beal
Morgan Kemp
Almas Jetha
Onelia Giarratano
Leon Sulmanis

And many, many others, unnamed by their choice, who gave kind and generous donations through the fundraising events and in other ways..........

<u>Thank you all from the bottom of my heart!</u>

APPENDIX 1

The wording for my GoFundme page:

Help Save Our Dad – Martyn Hopkins

"Anyone can be a father but it takes someone special to be a daddy"

Our Dad is tremendously special. He has always been there for us as a loving father, supporting our family in every part of our lives. He is honest, wise, he works hard, he is a good friend, he makes us laugh, he sees the best in people and importantly, he loves life!

He has worked so very hard in his life to provide for us, he has always been a gentle, positive and entertaining person – always handy with a joke or a ditty to bring a smile to your face. He has taught us excellent values and has always cheered us on for all our accomplishments.

....If a man's success is measured by how much his children love him, he is the most successful man ever. .....

You never imagine you may face losing someone so special to you…

In June 2018, Dad started to feel unwell and, thinking it was a water infection, went to the doctor for antibiotics. Shortly afterwards, blood tests revealed a PSA score of 441 indicating a problem – the doctor arranged for him to see a consultant.

After the consultant examined him, he was certain it was cancer. After having scans, we received the news that he had prostate cancer which had spread to his lymph nodes, pelvis and spine.

The consultants advised dad that they couldn't cure this; they could only buy him time – initially we were told 5-10 years, but following a biopsy, it was revealed that he has a rare sub-type of cancer (Ductal Adenocarcinoma) which is unusually aggressive, leaving us with the

Prognosis of 3-5 years.

As this type of cancer affects so few people, there is very little research into it, resulting in few and uncertain options for sufferers of it.

Treatment via the NHS consists only of chemotherapy and hormone treatment, but it is known that these therapies are less effective against Ductal Adenocarcinoma and generate potentially horrible side effects for very little time gain.

Dad researched treatments available elsewhere and came across a type of Immunotherapy offered in Beijing, where cells are manipulated to make them directly fight the cancer cells and turn the body's own immune system against the cancer. Whilst this is a new treatment, it is not without scientific backing – even the NHS is starting to use it but only for children with very advanced Leukaemia when all other treatments have failed.

Also available in Beijing is a treatment called Cryotherapy, which consists of inserting probes into the cancer tumour and alternates between deep freezing and super heating the tumour, until it dies. The Immunotherapy is then used to mop up any residual cancer cells and deal with the bone cancer.

Whilst there are no guarantees, the prognosis is a long-term remission and offers more hope than is available from treatments in the UK.

(These treatments are available in places in Europe but at very Significantly higher cost).

As it is, the treatment is going to cost £40,000 – a cost out of our league.

We want to work together to raise the money for Dad to be able to have his treatment in Beijing to give him a better quality of life and to give us a lot more time with him. We have to act fast as the longer we leave Dad untreated, the more the cancer can spread! As ever with cancer, time is not on our side.

We have set up this page and ask please that you help us by donating to our cause. We will also be arranging other fundraising activities along the way that you may be able to get involved in. Any additional funds raised over what we need will be donated to Prostate Cancer UK for further research into the treatment and cure of Prostate Cancer.

Thank you for taking the time to read this page – any help is gratefully and humbly received. Even sharing this page with friends, who you know will be interested, will help us so much!

Please help us save our daddy.

APPENDIX 2

Thanks to Sheena's foresight, we took with us the following items of food:

NIDO dried Milk large tin
Dried egg powder
Porridge Oats
Knorr dried chicken soup
Dried vegetables
Dry pasta
Bag of flour
Packets of Angel Delight
Cheese
Butter
Tea bags
Coffee in a jar
Hot chocolate sachets
McVities Digestives x 2 large packets.
Big bars of chocolate.
Salt and Pepper
Small pot of jam
Some packets of fruit and mint sweets.

These items were selected mostly because of their weight saving advantages, but we sacrificed some weight and space from our luggage allowance on the basis that we didn't know what we would find in China. Looking back, it was a wise move to have things that are so familiar with you, not least because western things, if you can find them, can be very expensive.

This list was supplemented by the bread and cakes we bought and a couple of trips to the Bon Marche supermarket in Beijing as well as the restaurant trips and takeaways organised by Cathy.

We also bought fresh fruit from local shops which was both good quality and very cheap.

We lived very well on this.

FOOTNOTE – APRIL 2021

I had a full body NHS CT scan in December 2020 during the Covid 19 pandemic. In a subsequent telephone consultation with my Oncologist she advised me that it was "good news". I could hardly wait….. she told me that there is no sign of cancer anywhere not primary or secondary cancers. My lymph nodes appear to be normal and even better news – where the cancer had been in my L5 vertebra but had gone leaving cavities, the bone is regenerating and closing the cavities!

Blood tests taken concurrently, also showed normal results and so no concerns there either.

Please bear in mind that this was two and a half years into a three to five years prognosis – and now there is no cancer at all.

I am still taking the three monthly Prostap injections as advised by both my Chinese and British Oncologists and unless and until something new and better comes along, it seems likely I will be on those permanently.

I suffer with back pain as a result of the damage caused by the cancer in my spine and as mentioned, Dr Dhu advised that this will be permanent. I am also awaiting a hip replacement as a result of severe Osteo Arthritis almost certainly caused, according to my Orthopaedic Surgeon, by the cancer.

I am not complaining – merely telling you, in a spirit of openness, how I now am – at time of writing, now almost three years from diagnosis in April 2021. To me, it is a price well worth paying as I feel generally very well.